Managing Patients' Organizations to Improve Healthcare:

Emerging Research and Opportunities

Francesca Costanza
University LUMSA, Palermo, Italy

A volume in the Advances in Healthcare Information Systems and Administration (AHISA) Book Series

IGI Global
DISSEMINATOR OF KNOWLEDGE

Published in the United States of America by
IGI Global
Medical Information Science Reference (an imprint of IGI Global)
701 E. Chocolate Avenue
Hershey PA, USA 17033
Tel: 717-533-8845
Fax: 717-533-8661
E-mail: cust@igi-global.com
Web site: http://www.igi-global.com

Library of Congress Cataloging-in-Publication Data

Names: Costanza, Francesca, 1982- author.
Title: Managing patients' organizations to improve healthcare : emerging research and opportunities / by Francesca Costanza.
Description: Hershey, PA : Medical Information Science Reference, [2020] | Includes bibliographical references and index. | Summary: "This book investigates the phenomenon of patient organizations looking at different dimensions (social, economic, managerial) from a multi-stakeholder perspective"-- Provided by publisher.
Identifiers: LCCN 2019041705 (print) | LCCN 2019041706 (ebook) | ISBN 9781799826538 (h/c) | ISBN 9781799826545 (eISBN)
Subjects: MESH: Patient Advocacy | Self-Help Groups | Patient Participation | Health Policy | Delivery of Health Care | Europe
Classification: LCC R727.45 (print) | LCC R727.45 (ebook) | NLM W 85.4 | DDC 362.1--dc23
LC record available at https://lccn.loc.gov/2019041705
LC ebook record available at https://lccn.loc.gov/2019041706

This book is published in the IGI Global book series Advances in Healthcare Information Systems and Administration (AHISA) (ISSN: 2328-1243; eISSN: 2328-126X)

British Cataloguing in Publication Data
A Cataloguing in Publication record for this book is available from the British Library.

Advances in Healthcare Information Systems and Administration (AHISA) Book Series

ISSN:2328-1243
EISSN:2328-126X

Editor-in-Chief: Anastasius Moumtzoglou, Hellenic Society for Quality & Safety in Healthcare and P. & A. Kyriakou Children's Hospital, Greece

MISSION

The **Advances in Healthcare Information Systems and Administration (AHISA) Book Series** aims to provide a channel for international researchers to progress the field of study on technology and its implications on healthcare and health information systems. With the growing focus on healthcare and the importance of enhancing this industry to tend to the expanding population, the book series seeks to accelerate the awareness of technological advancements of health information systems and expand awareness and implementation.

Driven by advancing technologies and their clinical applications, the emerging field of health information systems and informatics is still searching for coherent directing frameworks to advance health care and clinical practices and research. Conducting research in these areas is both promising and challenging due to a host of factors, including rapidly evolving technologies and their application complexity. At the same time, organizational issues, including technology adoption, diffusion and acceptance as well as cost benefits and cost effectiveness of advancing health information systems and informatics applications as innovative forms of investment in healthcare are gaining attention as well. **AHISA** addresses these concepts and critical issues.

COVERAGE

- IT Applications in Health Organizations and Practices
- Role of informatics specialists
- Rehabilitative Technologies
- Pharmaceutical and Home Healthcare Informatics
- IS in Healthcare
- Decision Support Systems
- IT Applications in Physical Therapeutic Treatments
- Medical Informatics
- Virtual health technologies
- Measurements and Impact of HISA on Public and Social Policy

IGI Global is currently accepting manuscripts for publication within this series. To submit a proposal for a volume in this series, please contact our Acquisition Editors at Acquisitions@igi-global.com or visit: http://www.igi-global.com/publish/.

The Advances in Healthcare Information Systems and Administration (AHISA) Book Series (ISSN 2328-1243) is published by IGI Global, 701 E. Chocolate Avenue, Hershey, PA 17033-1240, USA, www.igi-global.com. This series is composed of titles available for purchase individually; each title is edited to be contextually exclusive from any other title within the series. For pricing and ordering information please visit http://www.igi-global.com/book-series/advances-healthcare-information-systems-administration/37156. Postmaster: Send all address changes to above address.

Titles in this Series

For a list of additional titles in this series, please visit:
https://www.igi-global.com/book-series/advances-healthcare-information-systems-administration/37156

Handbook of Research on Optimizing Healthcare Management Techniques
Nilmini Wickramasinghe (Swinburne University of Technology, Australia & Epworth HealthCare, Australia)
Medical Information Science Reference • © 2020 • 431pp • H/C (ISBN: 9781799813712) • US $365.00

Theory and Practice of Business Intelligence in Healthcare
Jiban Khuntia (University of Colorado, Denver, USA) Xue Ning (University of Colorado, Denver, USA) and Mohan Tanniru (Oakland University, USA)
Medical Information Science Reference • © 2020 • 322pp • H/C (ISBN: 9781799823100) • US $245.00

Smart Medical Data Sensing and IoT Systems Design in Healthcare
Chinmay Chakraborty (Birla Institute of Technology, India)
Medical Information Science Reference • © 2020 • 288pp • H/C (ISBN: 9781799802617) • US $275.00

Emerging Trends and Innovations in Privacy and Health Information Management
Cristina Albuquerque (University of Coimbra, Portugal)
Medical Information Science Reference • © 2019 • 376pp • H/C (ISBN: 9781522584704) • US $275.00

Mobile Health Applications for Quality Healthcare Delivery
Anastasius Moumtzoglou (P&A Kyriakou Children's Hospital, Greece)
Medical Information Science Reference • © 2019 • 327pp • H/C (ISBN: 9781522580218) • US $265.00

Intelligent Systems for Healthcare Management and Delivery
Nardjes Bouchemal (University Center of Mila, Algeria)
Medical Information Science Reference • © 2019 • 377pp • H/C (ISBN: 9781522570714) • US $245.00

For an entire list of titles in this series, please visit:
https://www.igi-global.com/book-series/advances-healthcare-information-systems-administration/37156

IGI Global
DISSEMINATOR OF KNOWLEDGE

701 East Chocolate Avenue, Hershey, PA 17033, USA
Tel: 717-533-8845 x100 • Fax: 717-533-8661
E-Mail: cust@igi-global.com • www.igi-global.com

Table of Contents

Preface

Today's healthcare challenges regard the recognition of a patient-centered model, based on shared decision-making between patients and professionals, and the implementation of a patient co-created healthcare, where patients play the twofold role of customers and healthcare co-creators. In order to formulate quality decisions and to effectively contribute to the healthcare process, patients must be lay experts. The role of patients' organizations in education and capacity building is due to the fact that they aggregate many interacting voices, skills, values, preferences and ideas, so that the collective knowledge they are able to create is wider than the simple sum of individual contributions. Beside the educational role to patients, patient organizations can enhance physicians' skills to incorporate patients' perspective in the clinical practice, allowing a virtuous mix of evidence-based medicine and patient-centeredness.

Educated and empowered patients can collaborate with healthcare operators and providers to receive the best possible care, co-designing services and processes and even providing voluntary administrative work in the hospital lanes. Participating in steering committees and other institutional tables, patients' representatives can contribute to policy making and implementation at any stage of the policy making processes. They can also provide invaluable inputs to innovation processes, partnering public and private researches. The digital revolution poses new challenges for patients' participation in the healthcare processes, by giving patients the opportunity to be part of peer communities helping each other, sharing health data and information, communicating with doctors about their health conditions, obtaining key information about symptoms, treatments, experimental trials.

Despite the massive scientific and policy literature about the beneficial impact of patient engagement in healthcare provision, patient-centeredness is still far from being fully applied. The validity of patient organizations' work, although generally recognized, is undermined by external and internal issues:

externally, scarce social recognition and legislative attention to their role, internally, lacking managerial competencies and performance management skills and tools. This book has the double purpose to raise scientific and policy awareness about the contribution of patients' organizations in the healthcare process within regulatory authorities, public and healthcare managers, and to improve patient' managers and healthcare professionals' skills for more efficient and effective processes of care.

In order to pursue this scope, the book undertakes a comprehensive analysis of patient organizations' contribution to healthcare quality, putting together relevant scientific, policy and professional literature in a systematic way, and proceeding from a macro to a micro level. At the beginning chapter, patients' organizations are defined and introduced; then, each remaining chapter deals with a different facet of the theme: patient-aided policy making, patients' contributions to health delivery processes, skills and knowledge for patient organizations' management, dynamic models to support patient managers' decision making. Even though there currently exist many policy reports, patient organizations' communication materials and popular publications about the topic, there is a lack of scientific publications addressing it with such systemic, inter-institutional and multi-dimensional perspective.

In the first chapter, patients' organizations are described in general terms and in relation to patient-centeredness and patient empowerment. Then their activities are categorized by mean of an analytical framework combining territorial dimension (local, regional, national, international) and the focus of action (single disease or area of diseases, or several diseases from different areas). It emerges a taxonomy of four main typologies of patients' organizations.

The second chapter proposes an analysis of the patient advocacy's role within the policy making process. At first, the participation of patients in policy making through their representatives sitting at institutional working tables is framed in public management and administration theory. Switching from bureaucratic and purely managerialist approaches, New Public Governance, outcome-based and relational in nature, is considered a suitable theoretical foundation in which to comprehend the contributions of patients' organizations to the public policy discourse. Then, a feedback perspective on interactive policy making highlights potential policy cycles in pace with the patient inputs at each policy step. This chapter is relevant at current times of reflection on how to adapt healthcare systems to patients' needs and preference. According to the 2017 Report of European Patients Forum, entitled the *Added Value of Patient Organizations*, patients' participation in EU health policies is a reality, but the legislative landscape is still lacking and far from allowing a full disclosure of patients' potential. Indeed, despite national initiatives, patients' organizations are not provided with a clear EU legislative mandate including systematic reference to them in health policymaking.

In the third chapter, it is investigated how patient organizations can boost the delivery of healthcare. Such chapter, grounded in literature about co-creation, focuses two specific areas of patients' participation: education and aiding of R&D processes. There emerges a central role of patients' organizations in facilitating communication processes between several stakeholders, and differentiated contributions to innovation processes depending on the research's typologies, stages of research and level of patient expertise.

The fourth chapter makes an ample review of key requirements for effective patient organizations' management. Two are the key original research outputs of the chapter: the so-called 'antenna skill framework' and a business model canvas tailored to patients' organizations. The 'antenna skill framework' is a visual and practical illustration summarizing the necessary knowledge and skills for patient organizations' management. The key element of the structure is a generic patients' organization, which is represented as an antenna progressively picking up many kinds of knowledge and/or skills: about the institutional framework (and its sub-systems) in which the patients' organization is embedded, disease-related, technical and managerial knowledge and skills. The business model canvas tailored to patients' organizations builds on a business tool generally used for describing for-profit business models, and proposes a blended framework, mixing third-party funded enterprise models and social business models.

In the fifth chapter, the investigation targets the potential of system dynamics (or SD) modelling for patients' organizations. The choice of a simulation methodology to deal with patient-aided healthcare is because patients' organizations, beyond the 'physiological complexity' faced by other NGOs, must deal with the complexity of the healthcare sector in which they act. The chapter introduces key properties of complex systems like the healthcare one, and then motivates the suitability of system dynamics. It describes the building blocks of the methodology and sketches possible qualitative and quantitative modelling paths. Then it proposes a literature on previous applications to healthcare, distinguishing macro and micro modelling and identifying previous SD modelling efforts which have incorporated patient characteristics and perspective. Even though SD was successfully applied to many and differentiated healthcare issues, few models consider patients' characteristics and perspective, and none of them specifically deals with patients' organizations. Thus, it is descriptively outlined a research filling this gap in literature and depicting the outcome of patient organizations' participation in healthcare.

The sixth chapter proposes an original application of system dynamics, to frame the relationships between healthcare, patient organization's management and patient co-created healthcare. Based on an Italian case study, the methodological approach uses synergistically performance management and system dynamics. The chapter has the merit to both explain how to design the model and to show, step by step, the modelling outcomes: process maps, performance-based frameworks, stock-and-flow structures, feedback diagrams and quantitative simulations to undertake what-if analyses and ultimately to support decision-making. The dynamic performance management modelling approach means to bring a positive and a normative relevance, by forcing actors and decision makers to adopt a common view about the healthcare process, thereby contributing to better outputs and outcomes of care.

Overall, inputs, insights and ideas from this book could be tailored, with proper adaptations, to any type of patients' organizations, operating in different contexts and healthcare spheres. The policy reports cited in this book, mainly European and United States', are not meant to limit the validity of the analyses within specific territorial borders. On the contrary, in the author's view, since such reports deal with issues and processes in wide and general terms, they can be considered, together with relevant scientific literature, as valuable reference sources to drive some analyses enclosed in this work. The last chapter, even bearing in mind a specific case and requiring further research developments, could be easily scaled, with opportune adjustments, to another patients' organization.

This book is suitable for regulatory authorities and researchers in the fields of public management, healthcare management, social studies and third sector management. It is also meant to be to useful to patient organizations' managers to improve their skills and awareness, and to healthcare professionals and managers to promote more efficient and effective processes of care. Finally, this publication will also be helpful to inspire further research by post-graduate students interested in public management, healthcare management, social studies and third sector management.

Francesca Costanza

Acknowledgment

For the writing of this book the author did not received any fund or compensation and declares no conflict of interests. The first four chapters are mainly based on scientific and policy literature review and analysis, with the use of selected policy reports (in particular, elapsed within the European contexts), as leading frameworks because of their wide, general and informative connotations. The research methodology, presented in Chapter 5 and 6 and routed to system dynamics modelling in combination with performance management, was learned during author's PhD, an international program specialized in 'Model-based Public Policies Planning and Control', organized by University of Palermo (Italy), University of Bergen (Norway) and University of Nijmegen (The Netherlands).

Some concepts and issues reported in Chapter 6, together with the enclosed case study, are based on an author's research project, conducted in collaboration with the Sicilian Healthcare Department and ATTA, a patient association dealing with thyroid cancer management. However, this book only reflects the author's ideas and thoughts.

Chapter 1
The Patient-Centered Model and the Diffusion of Patients' Organizations

ABSTRACT

Healthcare management recognizes the importance of a patient-centered model whereas decision-making takes place pursuing social value, and empowered patients collaborate with healthcare operators in order to receive the best possible care. In this regard, patients' organizations are social groups taking care of patients' interests along several dimensions. This chapter introduces the phenomenon of patients' organizations and briefly describes the possible roles they can play within healthcare, both at macro and micro levels. The chapter organization is as follows: the background section introduces the importance of patient empowerment and describe the patient-centered healthcare model in general terms and as far as hospital organizational implications are concerned. It is followed by the definition of patients' organizations and a brief description of their diffusion. The chapter continues with a section about the social roles of patients' organizations, also considering the challenges posed by the digital transformation. It ends with conclusions and future research directions.

DOI: 10.4018/978-1-7998-2653-8.ch001

BACKGROUND

In the last decades, the definition of healthcare quality has evolved to take into consideration not just clinical outcomes but also patients' personal needs (Berghout *et al.*, 2015; Luxford *et al.*, 2011; Sepucha *et al.*, 2004). Such trend can be summarized by the affirmation of the 'patient-centered' care (Pelzang, 2010; Mead & Bower, 2000, 2002; Lawrence & Kinn 2012; World Health Organization, 2007), a model of healthcare provision characterized by respect and responsiveness of *individual patient preferences, needs, and values and ensuring that patient values guide all clinical decisions* (Institute of Medicine [IOM], 2001).

The introduction of the term in the medical field is ascribable to Balint (1957), whose research has progressively inspired medical and healthcare management literature, reporting the need for a shift from the traditional, paternalistic and professional/provider-focused approach to an egalitarian and patient-focused one. The results of this process are relevant healthcare improvements, especially on clinical outcomes, patient satisfaction, equity and efficiency (Arora *et al.*, 2009; Ford-Gilboe *et al.*, 2018; Prag *et al.*, 2017; Rathert *et al.*, 2013; Stewart, *et al.*, 2000; Street *et al.*, 2009). For these reasons, policy makers all over the world have included patient-centeredness within their agendas (Selby & Lipstein, 2014; Santana *et al.*, 2017).

At the same time, new tools and indicators have been developed to measure healthcare quality from the patient's perspective (Epstein & Street, 2011; Sawyer *et al.*, 2014; Sepucha *et al.*, 2004). In addition, the patient-centered care, called *partnership approach* by Cooper *et al.*, (2016), can be related to the person-centered model (Santana *et al.*, 2017) including also people not directly affected by illnesses but involved in the process of care, e.g. families and caregivers.

The core of the patient centered approach is its multi-dimensionality; according to the Picker Institute (Gerteis *et al.*, 1993), eight dimensions identify patient-centered care:

1. respect for patient preferences, values and expressed needs;
2. information, education and communication;
3. coordination and integration of care and services;
4. emotional support;
5. physical comfort;
6. involvement of family and friends;

7. continuity and transition;
8. access to care and services.

Thus, patient-centered care builds on patient participation and involvement, creating a relationship between the patient and the healthcare professional (Ford-Gilboe *et al.*, 2018), with the aim to ensure access to care and services, and by this way physical comfort and emotional support. The core of healthcare patient-centeredness is the transformation of the relationship between patients and doctors, the latter switching from 'agents in the name of patients' to a partnering role, supporting health decisions without abdicating from their professional responsibilities (Amato, 2016). The advantages of the approach have been widely explored in literature. Indeed, many sources report about patient and physician satisfaction, patients' empowerment, reduction of the symptoms of severity, increase in healthcare systems' efficiency, cost and consultation's time reduction and medication adherence (Ford-Gilboe et a., 2018; Little *et al.*, 2001; Stewart *et al.*, 2000; Stewart *et al.*, 2003). Patient-centered care in hospitals has been pointed out as a determinant of health outcomes' improvements, in terms of survival, greater patient satisfaction and well-being (Rathert *et al.*, 2013).

However, some researchers suggest that the impact of patient-centered care is not directly on health outcomes but works indirectly through other factors, such as positive healthcare perceptions. In particular, the process of recovery from illness is favored when patients perceive to *find a common ground* with physicians (Stewart *et al.*, 2000). Thus, patients' engagement is crucial for the quality of the healthcare and it is associated to the trust in the provider (Dang *et al.*, 2017). At the same time, effective communication between patients and professionals is associated with reductions in healthcare resources' needs and costs (Rao *et al.*, 2007).

The benefits of the patient-centered model are not limited to the evidence of clinical outcomes; but it can also serve as a stimulator for improving performance management within organizations, with relevant consequences in terms of managerial models and processes (Forio *et al.*, 2018; Brodersen & Thorwid, 1997; Hurst, 1995; Isaac *et al.*, 2010; Charmel & Frampton, 2008; IOM, 2001; Luxford *et al.*, 2011).

Shifting to patient-centeredness means for hospitals to redesign their structures from functional to process-oriented (Vera & Kunz, 2007), *going beyond the professional bureaucracy* (Lega & De Pietro, 2005) and inefficiencies that characterizes the hospitals, traditionally divided into functional, self-referential departments grouping all the patients who require similar areas of expertise. In the traditional model, patient admissions into the hospital structures take place under individual specialist clinicians, who reason separately (with no or limited coordination) from the other functions within the same organization and decide to retain or transfer them to the care of other clinicians. The patient-centered hospital model aims to rethink the healthcare delivery by focusing on healthcare processes in pace with the needs of the patients.

The application of the patient-centered approach at an organizational level requires a cultural change to go *beyond mainstream frameworks for quality improvement based on clinical measurement and audit* and to adopt *a strategic organizational approach to patient focus* (Luxford *et al.*, 2011). This means to create an organization able to involve patients and to learn from their experience (Groene *et al.*, 2009; Davies & Cleary, 2005; Wensing *et al.*, 2003).

The implementation of patient-centeredness at organizational level requires a systemic, comprehensive approach (Davies *et al.*, 2008). Six influencing key-factors need to be considered for the purpose: engagement of the top leadership; a strategic vision clearly and constantly communicated to every member of the organization; involvement of patients and families at multiple levels; a supportive work environment for all employees; systematic measurement and feedback; the quality of the built environment; and supportive information technology (Shaller, 2007). According to the European Patient Forum, a patient-centered healthcare requires patient empowerment, which is *about building patient-driven care where the patient is not only at the center of their care, but they are the most important member of their care team* (European Patient Forum [EPF], 2018, p. 7).

In order to actively contribute to their healthcare journey (Epstein, 2011), patients should be experts (Epstein, 1995) and be able to judge proficiently the information provided by clinicians and other operators within the healthcare system. Since there no exist universally accepted tools to evaluate healthcare information, the expert patient cannot work in isolation, but must be included in a social dimension allowing an intersubjective validation of knowledge. *Expert patient cannot be the one that accept passively information, but the one contributing to the creation of information through dialogue* (Del Fiore, 2016, p.2). Patients need to be part of wider patients' communities, made of people open to share their knowledge and to recognize the value of individual experiences and competences (Del Fiore, 2016). In this regard, patients' organizations can be seen as organized aggregations and combinations of single patient inputs, able to create a collective intelligence, whose development is greater than the mere sum of its constituting parts (Weinberger, 2011).

The goal of this chapter is to introduce patient organizations' features and their possible roles within healthcare. In order to address the scope, after this background section about patient-centered health, there is a section defining patients' organizations and their development. Then the chapter makes a review about the social roles of patients' organizations and proposes an analytical framework to describe the main typologies. Conclusions and future research avenues will be following.

THE PATIENTS' ORGANIZATIONS

According to the European Medicines Agency (EMA) patients' organizations are *not-for profit organizations which are patient focused, and whereby patients and/or carers (the latter when patients are unable to represent themselves) represent a majority of members in governing bodies* (Sienkiewicz & Van Lingen, 2017).

Patients' organizations were born in the Fifties as self-help groups to give patients the opportunity to share experiences about their own diseases. They soon enriched their sphere of action by including the defense of excluded patients. Their social role has progressively grown, then in 1978 the Alma Ata declaration of World Health Organization (WHO, 1978) stated that people's participation in the planning and implementation of their own healthcare is at the same time a right and a duty.

Patient advocacy was triggered by activist initiatives regarding HIV/AIDS, promoted in the year period 1980-1990 (Girardi, 2016). Beside the foundation of the International Steering Committee for People with HIV/AIDS in 1986, transformed in the Global Network of People Living with HIV/AIDS in 1992 (Amato, 2016), it is worth to mention that the US activist movements, over the time, had pushed research mechanisms for a cure, even achieving the participation of some of their components in institutional tables. Epstein (1995) identified factors contributing to the credibility of the activists (lay experts) in those institutional mechanisms: to learn the medical language, to show representativeness able to involve HIV patients to experimental procedures, to respect both equity and scientific rigor in clinical trials.

A vivacious debate on finding commonalities in medical and social sciences started from the Harvard School of Medicine, where it was conceived the anthropologic approach to medicine (Good, 1993). In this stream, later researches focused narrative medicine (Charon, 2006), patients' engagement in the healthcare process (Coulter, 2011) and patient-reported outcomes (Greenhalgh *et al.* 2015; Bellini & Kubler, 2018; Mc Lean *et al.*, 2019). Some scholars (Hoffman *et al.*, 2014) argued that evidence-based medicine and shared decision making are not contradictory concepts; in fact, they are interdependent and should be equally pursued for a quality healthcare. The importance of patient-reported outcomes was progressively recognized by public and private institutions. In 2009 the US Department of Health and Human Services elapsed a *guidance for industry* to support the use of patient-reported outcomes measures for medical products' development. In 2010 it was possible to assist to the foundation of the Patient-Centered Outcome Research Institute (PCORI) in Washington, with the scope to contribute to healthcare processes more patient-involving and informing.

In the European context, the process of EU integration started to affect national healthcare policies. Indeed, the Maastricht Treaty (1992) encouraged cooperation between Member States in the field of public health. This fact had two consequences: on the one hand, patients' organizations operating within the same disease areas, looked for a better social recognition and decided to merge in national bodies. On the other side, national patients' groups were induced to create alliances and synergies to work together at a European level. Few years later, the Amsterdam Treaty (1997) affirmed the importance for the European Union's policy making and implementation, to ensure high levels of human health protection, the urge to improve public health, as well as illness prevention. Such figures progressively stimulated international cooperation between several European patient groups, which at the beginning of the 21th century (2003) established the European Patients Forum, European patient organization integrating several areas of diseases. Starting with 13 members, today it consists of 74 EU organizations specifically focusing certain diseases (EPF Impact Report, 2018). The role of this organization is to be interlocutor in policy making, giving voice to patients' issues within the EU institutions.

The rules established by the European Patient Forum (EPF) to include trustful national organizations under its umbrella, namely the criteria for EPF memberships, are the following:

- transparency: disclosure of funding resources and audited financial accounts;
- legitimacy: members should be registered in at least one of the EU Member States;

- democracy: each patient organization should have a governing body elected by their members (patients, caregivers or elected representatives);
- representativeness: pan-European disease-specific organizations should have own members in more than half of the EU States. National platforms should represent at least 10 different disease groups in order to be accepted as full members;
- accountability and consultation: statements and opinions should reflect the views and opinions of their memberships.

According to EPF Report 2017, it is not known the exact number of patients' organizations worldwide or in Europe, due to the complexity of the phenomenon. Indeed, as far as EU is concerned, some organizations only operate at a local, regional or inter-regional level, whilst other organizations are active at a State level and do not search for European cooperation.

THE SOCIAL ROLES OF PATIENTS' ORGANIZATIONS

The involvement of patients in a highly professionalized area like healthcare is due to the fact that, although not bringing clinical knowledge, they can become experts in their own conditions and are the only people who are present at all stages during the provision of care: from diagnosis to recovery (Rathert *et al.*, 2011). Especially in chronic and rare diseases, patients know things that many professionals may not know (Bovaird, 2007) and then through their representative organizations, they can contribute to social value.

In first approximation, the possible roles of patients' organizations can be summarized into two main categories: support in policy making and support in healthcare delivery. About the first contribution, in line with a networked governance approach (Stoker, 2006), patients as key-stakeholders within healthcare, can actively participate in the processes of policy making and development at any stage. Indeed, the patients' representatives can provide the perspective of services' end-users and by this way can guide public decisions through the identification of priorities and measures.

The support in healthcare delivery has many facets: on the one hand, patients' organizations are reference point for people affected by a certain disease or group of diseases. Receiving support by peers who previously passed through the same health condition can improve self-confidence and compliance to the treatments (Stewart *et al.*, 2000; 2003). It can also boost processes of healthcare literacy (Altin & Stock, 2015; Berkman *et al.*, 2011) and self-management education to the community. At the hospital and community care level, patient organizations can influence management structures and the healthcare delivery flows by mean of collaborative capacity building with hospital managers, physicians and nurses. In some cases, the volunteers fill administrative gaps along the diagnostic and therapeutic path, for example in the hospital lanes and ambulatories they collaborate with hospital staff in patients' welcoming and bureaucratic assistance.

Those activities are particularly relevant at current times of progressive reduction of public budgets assignments (Simou & Koutsogeorgou, 2014; Burke *et al.*, 2014), whereas the third sector is determinant (Simsa *et al.*, 2014), and in public healthcare could allow medical staffs to maintain adequate level of service. Finally, the value of patients' organizations can be envisaged into research and development processes, especially in the pharmaceutical sector (Geissler *et al.,* 2017). The core activities are data collection, co-design, development and monitoring of healthcare innovations. These mechanisms are enhanced by digital technologies that are transforming the healthcare systems all over the world.

The digital revolution, the development of online platforms and the continuous production of big data are furtherly empowering patients and promoting virtuous circles of value co-creation (Elg *et al.*, 2012; Galvagno, & Dalli, 2014) and sustainability (Faggini *et al.*, 2018) through many possible kinds of interactions within the healthcare sector: patient-patient, patient-doctor, doctor-doctor. Physician rating websites provide useful information about patient satisfaction and allow patients to select a physician according to other patients' reviews and narrative comments, as well as digital surveys (Emmert *et al.*, 2015). Some services can be partially provided by mean of internet applications, especially in case of barriers to treatment such as *limited perceived need for treatment, preference to independently manage problems, inadequate finances, time constraints, transportation or mobility challenges, poor access to providers, or concerns about privacy and stigma* (Andrad *et al.*, 2014, as cited by Hadjistavropoulos *et al.*, 2017, p. 332). In other cases the subscription to an online community of peers dealing with the same disease and related issues can be useful to be part to a wider network, where patients can get precious information to which otherwise they would not have had access, for example news about patients' recruitments for experimental trials (Tozzi & Gesualdo, 2017).

Then the usefulness of patients' online interactions can go beyond the expression of satisfaction. Systematic collection and use of data, like patient-prioritized clinical and quality-of-life outcome (EPF, 2018, p.7), favored by online communication and information provision, can lead to a proficient use of patients' insights to make faster diagnosis, to improve healthcare outcomes and to develop and evaluate healthcare products' prototypes in the early design stage (Groeneveld *et al.*, 2019). In order to take advantage of this opportunity, it is crucial the building of patients' trust. The latter requires the protection of personal data and the possibility for the patients, as co-owners of their own data, to participate into the decision-making processes on data sharing and usage.

Notwithstanding, the EPF impact report (2018) recognizes the importance of digital health for healthcare provision, since it *can enable care to be structured around a person's needs and preferences, improve the coordination of care and have more effective exchange of information between care professionals and patients* (p. 7). The report above also cites the results of an expert working group about the patients' perspective on digital health. Such study, based on a patient survey on electronic health records, declares optimistic patients' expectations about digital healthcare, in terms of: facilitation of chronic disease management, self-management and quality of life improvement, patient empowerment and involvement in the care process as equal partners with healthcare professionals, improvement of the adherence to treatments, promotion of patient (and family) centered care as opposed to disease-centered, better integration of healthcare.

TYPOLOGIES OF PATIENTS' ORGANIZATIONS: AN ANALYTICAL FRAMEWORK

Patients' organizations are a special subset of human-centric NGOs (Robert Madelin, as reported by Sienkiewicz & Van Lingen, 2017). They can be distinguished from other civil society organizations because of their attention to patients both in focus and in memberships. Indeed, the other NGOs work on behalf of a wider constituency or society, while the peculiarity of patients' organizations is to focus on the needs of patients with patient-related membership criteria: members of patients' organizations are often patients and their relatives or caregivers, who often work on a voluntary basis. Their potential impact on healthcare is strong because they have first-hand experiences and can channel the voice of those they represent (Sienkiewicz & Van Lingen, 2017).

There currently exist many kinds of patients' organizations. Considering the case of chronic illnesses, table 1 groups them along two different dimensions: the vertical one is the territorial sphere of action, ranging from local/regional up to national European or international. The horizontal dimension represents the focus of action. Starting from the left, the amplitude and variety of issues with which the patients' organizations aim to deal, grow from one single disease or area of diseases, up to several diseases from different areas.

In the first quadrant there are single organizations which are active at a regional or local level and deal with issues related to a specific disease (e.g. diabetes, multiple sclerosis, Alzheimer's, etc.), or several diseases pertaining to a certain area of diseases (for example, rare diseases, cancers, mental health conditions, etc…). In this case, the organizations are close to the community of patients, to whom they provide two types of peer-to-peer interventions. First, they share a practical knowledge about their disease: in this case, they do not substitute the function of physicians and psychologists, but, as expert of their own diseases, they can help people with a recent diagnosis to familiarize with their new condition, motivating them to undertake the healthcare steps in light of their peers' experiences. This way, patients face the challenges launched by their diseases not feeling alone but being part of a group of people who already passed through the same problems and learnt how to live with them. On the other hand, patients' organizations can promote direct interventions within the processes of healthcare provision for the people they represent. For example, they can voluntarily work in hospitals and community cares to facilitate the booking and acceptance phases, the relation with medical staff, the preparation of the medical records, the release of the discharge card, the recall for follow-up activities. These interventions can be particularly relevant at times of austerity, characterized by cuts in public healthcare budgets, so the third sector can play a relevant role in providing services that the limited amount of resources cannot allow.

In the second quadrant, there are single organizations active at a regional or local level, not focusing specific diseases but dealing with patients' cross-cutting issues. The proximity to the local community also in this case stimulates operational interventions. Such activities are similar to the ones reported in the first quadrant, with the only difference that they are not condition specific-focused: they rather reflect a practical knowledge of the regional/local healthcare systems, the general facilitation of the healthcare access, the provision of information about bureaucratic steps for healthcare, diagnosis and preventions, etc…

Table 1. Analytic framework for typologies of patients' organizations

MAIN FOCUS / **TERRITORIAL SPHERE OF ACTION**	**Single Diseases or Single Areas of Diseases**	**Several Diseases from Different Areas**
Regional or Local	(1) SINGLE ORGANIZATIONS FOCUSING CONDITION-SPECIFIC ISSUES AT A REGIONAL/LOCAL LEVEL - Peer-to-peer sharing of practical knowledge about the disease - Peer-to-peer condition-specific direct interventions in the healthcare provision for the community	(2) SINGLE ORGANIZATIONS FOCUSING PATIENTS' CROSS-CUTTING ISSUES AT A REGIONAL/LOCAL LEVEL - Peer-to-peer sharing of practical knowledge about the healthcare provision - Peer-to-peer general interventions in the healthcare for the community (access facilitation, providing information about bureaucratic steps for healthcare…)
National, European or International	(3) NATIONAL ORGANIZATIONS OR COALITIONS OF ORGANIZATIONS FOCUSING CONDITION-SPECIFIC ISSUES AT A NATIONAL, EUROPEAN OR INTERNATIONAL LEVEL - Specialized peer-to-peer exchange of knowledge, expertise and best practices - Sensitization of public opinion about specific diseases/areas of diseases - Influence of public policy for stimulating condition-specific interventions	(4) NATIONAL ORGANIZATIONS OR COALITIONS OF ORGANIZATIONS FOCUSING PATIENTS' CROSS-CUTTING ISSUES AT A NATIONAL, EUROPEAN OR INTERNATIONAL LEVEL - Representation of patients' interests in relation to other stakeholders - Influence of public policy for stimulating interventions about healthcare quality, structure of the healthcare system, accessibility, discrimination, etc…

Beside regional and local organizations there are national patients' organizations which, together with regional and local ones, can be part of wider organizations, coalitions of operators intervening at a national, European or international level. In the third quadrant there are national organizations focusing specific pathologies (or groups of pathologies), as well as coalitions of patients' organizations (operating at local, regional or national level), which are umbrella organizations. Their sphere of action can be national or supranational. The existence of a national body (in term of single operator or coalition of operators) favors the sharing of knowledge, expertise and best practices that could be replicated in other territorial contexts. The national organizations can also work for the sensitization of the public opinion about certain diseases through media campaigns for patients' social integration and fundraising. They can even influence the public policy making to address condition-specific issues, for example devoting budgets to prevention, care and research about such pathologies. Supranational disease-specific organizations enable national patients' organizations active in the same disease-area to compare situations between countries. For example, the EPF tracks for specific diseases the treatments and care available across Europe, promotes the transfer of good practices and monitors legislative developments at EU level (Sienkiewicz & Van Lingen, 2017).

In the last quadrant it is reported the case of national or supranational patients' organizations (in the form of single organization or coalition of organizations operating at national, regional or local level) not focusing specific pathologies or groups of pathologies, but integrating and representing the collective interest of all patients in a country or at a pan-European or international level. These organizations can take part to an inter-institutional dialogue with other stakeholders and can even intervene in the formulation and implementation of policy measures about the healthcare provision, on a national and supranational basis. Such organizations, working on cross-cutting issues (e.g. access to care, discrimination, structure of healthcare systems) related to the healthcare systems, enable disease-specific organizations to focus on their area of specialism. In EU, the most important supranational organization is the EPF, which works both at disease-specific level and at a general cross-cutting level. It includes national coalitions and pan-European disease-specific organizations. This means that local, regional and national disease-specific organizations are not eligible for EPF membership, but they can be members of national coalitions and European umbrella organizations that are members of EPF (Sienkiewicz & Van Lingen, 2017). Sometimes patients' organizations are not legally formalized and are based on the spontaneous formation of groups of people still aiming to provide a contribution to the quality of healthcare. These informal organizations are often considered as sub-groups within broader organizations or alliances and include also other stakeholders, like caregivers, healthcare professionals, scholars.

FUTURE RESEARCH DIRECTIONS

The chapter addressed in general terms the phenomenon of patients' organizations and made a hint of the possible roles they can play within healthcare. The content analysis performed on scientific publications and policy reports remarked the importance of patient-centeredness and engagement for the pursuing of a high-quality healthcare, as well as the contribution of the patients' organizations for the scope. The study also proposed an original analytical framework to create a taxonomy of patients' organizations and described the possible social roles of these actors. Next researches should deepen the analyses already conducted, focusing specific aspects, such case studies about patient participation in the healthcare policies' design and implementation and to the delivery of healthcare. Particularly important is to investigate the impact of digital health on each step of patients' involvement. These efforts should pair patients' consultation and participation with the engagement of other relevant stakeholders in the healthcare sectors, for example policy makers, regional or local healthcare authorities, hospital managers, administrative personnel, physicians and nurses. The inter-institutional perspective could help to foster a shared view of the causal tissue determining the healthcare performances and the value creation, thus allowing an effective patient-centeredness.

CONCLUSION

Traditional healthcare has focused its attention on clinical outcomes and physicians' perspective, neglecting the central role of patients and their organizations. Recent researches and applications have demonstrated that patient is not just a passive recipient of care, but it can be an active participant through the entire process of health service delivery. The chapter made a general description of several patient contributions to quality and effective healthcare. Such interventions go from the mere expression of satisfaction driving other patients' choices to the co-creation of products and services. The patients' organizations are based on patient-centeredness, which can also inspire organizational changes in hospitals and community care, with de-bureaucratization and redesign of structures from functional to process-oriented.

In line with this study, the main challenge for patients' organizations is the social recognition of patient expertise about their own condition and their crucial role, both at a macro and at a micro level. At a macro level, the consultation of patients' organizations can be useful tools to address public decision makers and to facilitate the identification of priorities. At a micro level, patient organizations' inputs and activities can provide peer to peer help, promote healthcare literacy, collaborate in service provision, and their insights can stimulate organizational and operational changes, improving healthcare performance management. Finally, the ongoing digital transformation, giving a general opportunity to structure services around people's personal needs and preferences, can furtherly boost patients' engagement, favor an effective exchange of information between care professionals and patients, and improve coordination mechanisms between healthcare actors.

REFERENCES

Altin, S. V., & Stock, S. (2015). Impact of health literacy, accessibility and coordination of care on patient's satisfaction with primary care in Germany. *BMC Family Practice*, *16*(1), 148–154. doi:10.118612875-015-0372-0 PMID:26492959

Amato, L. (2016). Empowerment e engagement del Cittadino. Alcune tappe recenti della crescita del ruolo dei cittadini nella sanità. *Forward – Pazienti*, *3*, 4-5.

Andrade, L. H., Alonso, J., Mneimneh, Z., Wells, J. E., Al-Hamzawi, A., Borges, G., ... De Graaf, R. (2014). Barriers to mental health treatment: Results from the WHO world mental health surveys. *Psychological Medicine*, *44*(6), 1303–1317. doi:10.1017/S0033291713001943 PMID:23931656

Arora, N. K., Weaver, K. E., Clayman, M. L., Oakley-Girvan, I., & Potosky, A. L. (2009). Physicians' decision-making style and psychosocial outcomes among cancer survivors. *Patient Education and Counseling*, *77*(3), 404–412. doi:10.1016/j.pec.2009.10.004 PMID:19892508

Ashish, K., Jha, M., & Orav, E. (2008). Patients' perception of hospital care in the United States. *The New England Journal of Medicine*, *359*(18), 1921–1931. doi:10.1056/NEJMsa0804116 PMID:18971493

Balint, M. (1957). *The Doctor, His Patient and the Illness*. London, UK: Pitman Medical. doi:10.1097/00000441-195711000-00018

Bellini, M., & Kubler, A. (2018). Health Literacy and Patient-Reported Outcomes. In *Optimizing Health Literacy for Improved Clinical Practices* (pp. 109–123). Hershey, PA: IGI Global. doi:10.4018/978-1-5225-4074-8.ch007

Berghout, M., Van Exel, J., Leensvaart, L., & Cramm, J. M. (2015). Healthcare professionals' views on patient centered care in hospitals. *BMC Health Services Research*, *15*(1), 385–397. doi:10.118612913-015-1049-z PMID:26373841

Berkman, N. D., Sheridan, S. L., Donahue, K. E., Halpern, D. J., & Crotty, K. (2011). Low Health Literacy and Health Outcomes: An Updated Systematic Review. *Annals of Internal Medicine*, *155*(2), 97–107. doi:10.7326/0003-4819-155-2-201107190-00005 PMID:21768583

Bovaird, T. (2007). Beyond Engagement and Participation: User and Community Coproduction of Public Services. *Public Administration Review*, *67*(5), 846–860. doi:10.1111/j.1540-6210.2007.00773.x

Brodersen, J., & Thorwid, J. (1997). Enabling sustainable change for healthcare in Stockholm. *The British Journal of Healthcare Computing & Information Management*, *14*(4), 23–26.

Burke, S., Thomas, S., Barry, S., & Keegan, C. (2014). Indicators of health system coverage and activity in Ireland during the economic crisis 2008–2014. From 'more with less' to 'less with less'. *Health Policy (Amsterdam)*, *117*(3), 275–278. doi:10.1016/j.healthpol.2014.07.001 PMID:25082466

Charmel, P., & Frampton, S. (2008). Building the business case for patient centered care. *Healthcare Financial Management*, *62*, 80–85. PMID:19097611

Charon, R. (2006). *Narrative Medicine. Honoring the Stories of Illness*. New York, NY: Oxford University Press.

Cooper, H., McMurray, A., Ward, L., & Connor, M. (2016). Implementing patient-centred care in the context of an integrated care program. *International Journal of Care Coordination*, *18*(4), 72–77. doi:10.1177/2053434516639336

Coulter, A. (2011). *Engaging Patients in Healthcare*. Maidenhead, UK: Open University Press - McGraw-Hill Education Europe.

Dang, B. N., Westbrook, R. A., Njue, S. M., & Giordano, T. P. (2017). Building trust and rapport early in the new doctor-patient relationship: A longitudinal qualitative study. *BMC Medical Education*, *17*(1), 32–41. doi:10.118612909-017-0868-5 PMID:28148254

Davies, E., & Cleary, P. D. (2005). Hearing the patient's voice? Factors affecting the use of patient survey data in quality improvement. *Quality & Safety in Health Care*, *14*(6), 428–432. doi:10.1136/qshc.2004.012955 PMID:16326789

Del Fiore, L. (2016). Antonella, Patrizia e la competenza da costruire insieme. Storie di partecipazione e coinvolgimento. *Forward – Pazienti*, *3*, 2-3.

Elg, M., Engström, J., Witell, L., & Poksinska, B. (2012). Co-creation and learning in health-care service development. *Journal of Service Management*, *23*(3), 328–343. doi:10.1108/09564231211248435

Emmert, M., Adelhardt, T., Sander, U., Wambach, V., & Lindenthal, J. (2015). A cross-sectional study assessing the association between online ratings and structural and quality of care measures: Results from two German physician rating websites. *BMC Health Services Research*, *15*(414), 1–9. PMID:26404452

Epstein, R. M., & Street, R. L. (2011). The Values and Value of Patient-Centered Care. *Annals of Family Medicine*, *9*(2), 100–103. doi:10.1370/afm.1239 PMID:21403134

Epstein, S. (1995). The Construction of Lay Expertise: AIDS Activism and the Forging of Credibility in the Reform of Clinical Trials. *Science, Technology & Human Values*, *20*(4), 408–437. doi:10.1177/016224399502000402 PMID:11653331

European Patients Forum. (2018). *Impact Report 2018*. Brussel: European Patients Forum.

Faggini, M., Cosimato, S., Nota, F. D., & Nota, G. (2018). Pursuing Sustainability for Healthcare through Digital Platforms. *Sustainability*, *11*(1), 165–179. doi:10.3390u11010165

Fiorio, C. V., Gorli, M., & Verzillo, S. (2018). Evaluating organizational change in healthcare: The patient-centered hospital model. *BMC Health Services Research*, *18*(1), 95–109. doi:10.118612913-018-2877-4 PMID:29422045

Ford-Gilboe, M., Wathen, C. N., Varcoe, C., Herbert, C., Jackson, B. E., Lavoie, C. J., ... Browne, A. J. (2018). How Equity-Oriented Healthcare Affects Health: Key Mechanisms and Implications for Primary Healthcare Practice and Policy. *The Milbank Quarterly*, *96*(4), 635–671. doi:10.1111/1468-0009.12349 PMID:30350420

Galvagno, M., & Dalli, D. (2014). Theory of value co-creation: A systematic literature review. *Journal of Service Theory and Practice*, *24*(6), 643–683.

Geissler, J., Ryll, B., Leto di Priolo, S., & Uhlenhopp, M. (2017). Improving Patient Involvement in Medicines Research and Development: A Practical Roadmap. *Therapeutic Innovation & Regulatory Science*, *51*(5), 1–8. doi:10.1177/2168479017706405 PMID:30231692

Gerteis, M., Edgman-Levitan, S., Walker, J. D., Stoke, D. M., Cleary, P. D., & Delbanco, T. L. (1993). What patients really want. *Health Management Quarterly*, *15*(3), 2–6. PMID:10129190

Girardi, E. (2016). Da vittime a esperti. L'impatto dell'attivismo per l'hiv sulla ricerca clinica. *Forward – Pazienti*, *3*, 4-5.

Good, B. J. (1993). *Medicine, rationality and experience: an anthropological perspective. Lewis Henry Morgan Lectures Series*. New York, NY: Cambridge University Press. doi:10.1017/CBO9780511811029

Greenhalgh, T., Snow, R., Ryan, S., Rees, S., & Salisbury, H. (2015). Six 'biases' against patients and carers in evidence-based medicine. *BMC Medicine*, *13*(1), 200–210. doi:10.118612916-015-0437-x PMID:26324223

Groene, O., Lombarts, M. J., Klazinga, N., Alonso, J., Thompson, A., & Sunol, R. (2009). Is patient-centredness in European hospitals related to existing quality improvement strategies? Analysis of a cross-sectional survey (Marquis study). *Quality & Safety in Health Care*, *18*(Suppl 1), 44–50. doi:10.1136/qshc.2008.029397 PMID:19188461

Groeneveld, B., Melles, M., Vehmeijer, S., Mathijssen, N., Dekkers, T., & Goossens, R. (2019). Developing digital applications for tailored communication in orthopaedics using a Research through Design approach. *Digital Health*, *5*, 1–14. doi:10.1177/2055207618824919 PMID:30719322

Hadjistavropoulos, H. D., Nugent, M. M., Dirkse, D., & Pugh, N. (2017). Implementation of internet-delivered cognitive behavior therapy within community mental health clinics: A process evaluation using the consolidated framework for implementation research. *BMC Psychiatry*, *17*(1), 331–345. doi:10.118612888-017-1496-7 PMID:28899365

Hoffman, T. C., Montori, V. M., & Del Mar, C. (2014). The Connection Between Evidence-Based Medicine and Shared Decision Making. *Journal of the American Medical Association*, *312*(13), 1295–1296. doi:10.1001/jama.2014.10186 PMID:25268434

Hurst, K. (1995). *Progress with Patient Focused Care in the United Kingdom*. Leeds, UK: NHS Executive.

Institute of Medicine. (2001). *Crossing the quality chasm: A new health system for the 21st century, report, Committee on Quality of Healthcare in America*. Washington, DC: National Academies Press.

Isaac, T., Zaslavsky, A., Cleary, P. D., & Landon, B. E. (2010). The Relationship between Patients' Perception of Care and Measures of Hospital Quality and Safety. *Health Services Research*, *45*(4), 1024–1040. doi:10.1111/j.1475-6773.2010.01122.x PMID:20528990

Lawrence, M., & Kinn, S. (2012). Defining and measuring patient-centred care: An example from a mixed-methods systematic review of the stroke literature. *Health Expectations*, *15*(3), 295–326. doi:10.1111/j.1369-7625.2011.00683.x PMID:21624025

Lega, F., & De Pietro, C. (2005). Converging patterns in hospital organization: Beyond the professional bureaucracy. *Health Policy (Amsterdam)*, *74*(3), 261–281. doi:10.1016/j.healthpol.2005.01.010 PMID:16226138

Little, P., Everitt, H., Williamson, I., Warner, G., Moore, M., Gould, C., ... Payne, S. (2001). Observational study of effect of patient centredness and positive approach on outcomes of general practice consultations. *British Medical Journal*, *323*(7318), 908–911. doi:10.1136/bmj.323.7318.908 PMID:11668137

Luxford, K., Safran, D. G., & Delbanco, T. (2011). Promoting patient-centered care: A qualitative study of facilitators and barriers in healthcare organizations with a reputation for improving the patient experience. *International Journal for Quality in Health Care*, *23*(5), 510–515. doi:10.1093/intqhc/mzr024 PMID:21586433

Mc Lean, K. A., Drake, T. M., Sgrò, A., Camilleri-Brennan, J., Knight, S. R., Ots, R., ... Harrison, E. M. (2019). The effect of liver transplantation on patient-centred outcomes: A propensity-scorematched analysis. *Transplant International*, *32*(8), 808–819. PMID:30793373

Mead, N., & Bower, P. (2000). Patient-centredness: A conceptual framework and review of the empirical literature. *Social Science & Medicine*, *51*(7), 1087–1110. doi:10.1016/S0277-9536(00)00098-8 PMID:11005395

Mead, N., & Bower, P. (2002). Patient-centred consultations and outcomes in primary care: A review of the literature. *Patient Education and Counseling*, *48*(1), 51–61. doi:10.1016/S0738-3991(02)00099-X PMID:12220750

Pelzang, R. (2010). Time to learn: Understanding patient-centred care. *British Journal of Nursing (Mark Allen Publishing)*, *19*(14), 912–917. doi:10.12968/bjon.2010.19.14.49050 PMID:20647984

Prag, P., Wittek, R., & Mills, M. C. (2017). The educational gradient in self-rated health in Europe: Does the doctor–patient relationship make a difference? *Acta Sociologica*, *60*(4), 325–341. doi:10.1177/0001699316670715

Rao, J. K., Anderson, L. A., Inui, T. S., & Frankel, R. M. (2007). Communication interventions make a difference in conversations between physicians and patients: A systematic review of the evidence. *Medical Care*, *45*(4), 340–349. doi:10.1097/01.mlr.0000254516.04961.d5 PMID:17496718

Rathert, C., Huddleston, N., & Pak, Y. (2011). Acute care patients discuss the patient role in patient safety. *Health Care Management Review*, *36*(2), 134–144. doi:10.1097/HMR.0b013e318208cd31 PMID:21317659

Rathert, C., Wyrwich, M. D., & Boren, S. A. (2013). Patient-centered care and outcomes a systematic review of the literature. *Medical Care Research and Review: MCRR*, *70*(4), 351–379. doi:10.1177/1077558712465774 PMID:23169897

Santana, M. J., Manalili, K., Jolley, R. J., Zelinsky, S., Quan, H., & Lu, M. (2017). How to practice person-centred care: A conceptual framework. *Health Expectations*, *21*(2), 429–440. doi:10.1111/hex.12640 PMID:29151269

Sawyer, S. M., Ambresin, A. E., Bennett, K. E., & Patton, G. C. (2014). A measurement framework for quality healthcare for adolescents in hospital. *The Journal of Adolescent Health*, *55*(4), 484–490. doi:10.1016/j.jadohealth.2014.01.023 PMID:24698286

Selby, J. V., & Lipstein, S. H. (2014). PCORI at 3 years. Progress, lessons, and plans. *The New England Journal of Medicine*, *370*(7), 592–595. doi:10.1056/NEJMp1313061 PMID:24521104

Sepucha, K. R., Fowler, F. J., Jr., & Mulley, A. G., Jr. (2004). Policy Support For Patient- Centered Care: The Need For Measurable Improvements In Decision Quality. *Health Affairs*, 54-62.

Shaller, D. (2007). *Patient-centered care: what does it take? Report for the Picker Institute and The Commonwealth Fund*. New York, NY: The Commonwealth Fund.

Sienkiewicz, D., & Van Lingen, C. (2017). *The Added Value of Patient Organisations, Report EPF European Patients Forum Work Program*. Brussels: European Patients Forum.

Simou, E., & Koutsogeorgou, E. (2014). Effects of the economic crisis on health and healthcare in Greece in the literature from 2009 to 2013: A systematic review. *Health Policy (Amsterdam), 115*(2-3), 111–119. doi:10.1016/j.healthpol.2014.02.002 PMID:24589039

Simsa, R., Rauscher, O., Schober, C., & Moder, C. (2014). *Impact. Methodological Guideline for Impact Assessment.* Working paper n. 01. Brussels: Seventh Framework Programme European Union.

Stewart, M., Brown, J. B., & Donner, A. (2000). The impact of patient-centered care on outcomes. *The Journal of Family Practice, 49*, 796–804. PMID:11032203

Stewart, M., Brown, J. B., Weston, W. W., & Freeman, T. R. (2003). *Patient-Centred Medicine: Transforming the Clinical Method* (2nd ed.). Radcliffe, UK: Radcliffe Medical Press.

Stoker, G. (2006). Public Value Management A New Narrative for Networked Governance? *American Review of Public Administration, 36*(1), 41–57. doi:10.1177/0275074005282583

Street, R. L. Jr, Makoul, G., Arora, N. K., & Epstein, R. M. (2009). How does communication heal? Pathways linking clinician-patient communication to health outcomes. *Patient Education and Counseling, 74*(3), 295–301. doi:10.1016/j.pec.2008.11.015 PMID:19150199

Tozzi, E., & Gesualdo, F. (2016). Salute partecipativa? La tecnologia digitale aiuta. *Forward – Pazienti, 3*, 22-23.

US Department of Health and Human Services. (2009). *Guidance for Industry Patient-Reported Outcome Measures: Use in Medical Product Development to Support Labeling Claims.* Washington, DC: US Department of Health and Human Services.

Vera, A., & Kuntz, L. (2007). Process-based organization design and hospital efficiency. *Health Care Management Review, 32*(1), 55–65. doi:10.1097/00004010-200701000-00008 PMID:17245203

Weinberger, D. (2011). *Too Big to Know: Rethinking Knowledge Now That the Facts Aren't the Facts, Experts Are Everywhere, and the Smartest Person in the Room.* New York, NY: Basic Books.

Wensing, M., Vingerhoets, E., & Grol, R. (2003). Feedback based on patient evaluations: A tool for quality improvement? *Patient Education and Counseling, 51*(2), 149–153. doi:10.1016/S0738-3991(02)00199-4 PMID:14572944

World Health Organization. (1978). *Alma-Ata Primary healthcare, Health for all series, n. 1.* Geneva: WHO Regional Office for Europe.

World Health Organization. (2007). People-centred healthcare: A policy framework. Geneva: World Health Organization.

ADDITIONAL READING

Hudon, C., Fortin, M., Haggerty, J. L., Lambert, M., & Poitras, M. (2011). Measuring Patients' Perceptions of Patient-Centered Care: A Systematic Review of Tools for Family Medicine. *Annals of Family Medicine, 9*(2), 155–164. doi:10.1370/afm.1226 PMID:21403143

Kane, P. M., Murtagh, F. E. M., Ryan, K., Mahon, N. G., McAdam, B., McQuillan, R., ... Daveson, B. A. (2015). The gap between policy and practice: A systematic review of patient-centred care interventions in chronic heart failure. *Health Fail Review, 20*(6), 673–687. doi:10.100710741-015-9508-5 PMID:26435042

Kuipers, S. J., Cramm, J. M., & Nieboer, A. P. (2019). The importance of patient-centered care and co-creation of care for satisfaction with care and physical and social well-being of patients with multi-morbidity in the primary care setting. *BMC Health Services Research, 19*(13), 1–9. PMID:30621688

Levinson, W., Lesser, C. S., & Epstein, R. M. (2010). Developing Physician Communication Skills For Patient-Centered Care. *Health Affairs, 29*(7), 1310–1318. doi:10.1377/hlthaff.2009.0450 PMID:20606179

McCaffrey, S. A., Chiauzzi, E., Chan, C., & Hoole, M. (2018). Understanding 'Good Healthcare' from the Patient's Perspective: Development of a Conceptual Model Using Group Concept Mapping. *The Patient-Centered Outcomes Research, 12*(1), 83–95. doi:10.100740271-018-0320-x

KEY TERMS AND DEFINITIONS

Chronic Conditions or Chronic Diseases: Human health conditions enduring the whole person's life or for a long-lasting period of time (usually more than three months). They usually affect multiple areas of the body and are not fully responsive to treatment. Examples of chronic diseases are arthritis, asthma, cancer. Chronic conditions are usually distinguished from the acute ones.

Digital Health: A multidisciplinary domain consisting on the use of information and communication technologies to enhance healthcare processes. The scope is the development of interconnected health systems able to manage illnesses and health risks, and to promote health and wellbeing through computational technologies and smart devices. It includes several applications and services, such as telemedicine, web-based analysis, email, smartphone applications, text messages, wearable devices, social media. These figures favor communication mechanisms between many healthcare stakeholders (patients, clinicians, researchers and scientists, engineers, social scientist, public health's decision makers, data managers).

Inter-Institutional Perspective: Approach of policy analysis and design which takes into consideration the view of several institutional actors about a certain theme or issue. This implies to cross the boundaries of single organizations and to consider cross-cutting issues and processes involving the contribution of several stakeholders to public value creation.

Patient Organizations: Not-for profit organizations which are patient-focused, and whereby patients and caregivers represent most of members in governing bodies. Their key characteristics are transparency in the sources of funding, legitimacy, democracy rules in their governing bodies, representativeness at national, international and local level, presence of accountability and consultation procedures.

Patient-Centered Model: Model of healthcare provision characterized by respect and responsiveness of individual patients' preferences and needs, ensuring that patient values guide all clinical decisions. It requires a shift from a traditional approach, which is paternalistic and focused on professionals and providers, to a new egalitarian approach, focused on patients, their families and caregivers.

Process-Oriented Organizations: Organizations whose structures and performance measurement systems are based on processes rather than functions. They formally design, document and monitor operational processes and their interrelations, identifying for each process a process owner (i.e., a responsible manager). A process-oriented organization is also characterized by a culture of teamwork and collaboration, change management, and focus on customers (patients in the case of healthcare organizations).

Chapter 2
Patient Advocacy and the Policy Making Process

ABSTRACT

Recent developments in the policy-making literature and practice have highlighted the growing role of patient advocacy, that is, the participation of patients in policy making through the presence of their representatives at institutional working tables. This chapter has a twofold aim: (1) to frame the activity of patient organizations' advocacy into the public management and administration theory and (2) to describe how patients' organizations can participate to the public policy making from an operational point of view. The chapter starts by providing background information about patient advocacy. Then it introduces the core literature streams of public management and administration. Finally, a feedback analysis shows possible policy cycles linking patient-aided steps of interactive policy making.

BACKGROUND

Patients' organizations are non-profit entities made up of a group of voluntary people, aggregated to pursue common purposes: to represent patients, to provide them practical information for a better management of their own pathologies, to support patients and their entourage (families and caregivers), to organize public campaigns promoting awareness about the diseases, to collaborate with health facilities and institutions, and to carry out advocacy activities. The latter function, representing the main focus of the present chapter, requires

DOI: 10.4018/978-1-7998-2653-8.ch002

providing a definition of patient advocacy. Indeed, patient organizations are no just spokespersons for patients' needs but key stakeholders, empowered and informed, active participants in the health policy choices. Sometimes the term 'advocacy' is used to indicate the concept of any activity carried on by patients' organizations. It is not the case of this chapter, which instead uses this word by recalling its Latin etymology ('to add a voice') and thus accepts the meaning *to promote and defend the patients' cause by bringing their needs to the policy makers* (Aloe & De Stefano, 2017).

Patient advocacy builds on patient empowerment and engagement, two relevant concepts influencing each other. Empowerment is a social process occurring when people, organizations and communities acquire expertise on their own lives, gain mastery of their affairs, change their social and political environment, and improve equity and quality of life (Wallerstein, 2006; Rappaport, 1987).

In the healthcare sector, it translates into people's conscious participation in the management of healthcare. Empowerment can be seen at an individual or at a community level. Individual empowerment means people's feeling of a sense of control over their lives (Woodal *et al.,* 2010)., which research positively links to mental and physical health (Wallerstein, 1992; 2003). However, individual empowerment is limited because it does not consider the wider environmental influences on people's health (Woodal *et al.,* 2010). Thus, it is the case to complement the individual's notion to the collective one, i.e. the community empowerment, able to overcome individual interests of skill formation, and to create communities that can support social changes by mean of partnerships, participation and collective action (Wallerstein, 2006).

Thus, it becomes necessary to valorize patients' expertise about their own illnesses and the necessary know-how to coexist with them, at the same time increasing individual and collective patients' knowledge and skills. The latter can only happen through patients' engagement, i.e. involving them in decisions regarding planning, management and evaluation of healthcare services, and thereby contributing to the sustainability of the health system (Balduzzi, 2009). Indeed, patient advocacy implies the use of strategic information to change public policies and allocative decisions that have a direct impact on people's lives, as well as to direct collective and individual behaviors to the improvement of individuals and communities' health (Aloe & De Stefano, 2017).

The present chapter has the following goals:

1. to frame the activity of patient organizations' advocacy into the public management and administration theory;
2. to describe how patient organizations can participate in the public policy making from an operational point of view.

According to the above scopes, after this background section, the chapter introduces the core literature streams of public management and administration and proposes a feedback analysis showing possible operational cycles within patient-aided interactive policy steps. Finally, conclusions and future research avenues are provided.

FRAMING PATIENT ADVOCACY INTO PUBLIC MANAGEMENT THEORIES

Nowadays patients' participation in public policies is acknowledged as a possible way to reach effective decision making (Del Fiore, 2016). A recent example of this involvement can be retrieved in the European Union, where the help of patients was called to favour the implementation of the Directive on Cross-border Healthcare at Member State level. Such regulation was legislated in 2011 and expected to be put in action by States within the next biennial. Then, patients' organisations helped policymakers to assess the impact of the Directive, provided feedbacks to EU institutions about the operational ways it was implemented by national governments, and made policy recommendations for improvements and adjustments (Sienkiewicz & Van Lingen, 2017, p. 10).

However, the role of patients' organizations as interlocutors for policy and pharmaceutical industry is delicate, because it postulates patient organizations' credibility and capacity to preserve its decisional independency and transparency (Del Fiore, 2016). Furthermore, it can be envisaged an issue of timeliness of involvement in the policy building. As in the example mentioned above, patients are prominently required in the last phases of the policy process (approving and regulatory phases), whilst their perspective is usually overlooked in the upward stages, for example in research priority setting, where they can bring an even wider added value (Liberati, 2011).

The potential patients' contribution to healthcare policy can be better understood in light of the main streams of public management and administration theories. Indeed, according to the author, knowing the characteristics of the three 'umbrella concepts' of traditional Public Administration, New Public Management and New Public Governance can provide some lenses to understand the foundations of patients' advocacy.

The first theoretical branch is based on the Weberian, traditional, bureaucracy (Weber, 1922). This is an administration model basing its legitimization and rationality on legal power and hierarchal mechanisms. Bureaucracy postulates quick responses to public needs through rigid written rules and procedures, supposed to allow precision and behavioral uniformity. Another feature of bureaucracy is the net definition of borders between the administrative (or bureaucratic) and political spheres, the first setting public institutions' goals, the second in charge of their neutral execution (Wilson, 1887). For long time the bureaucratic model has been applied to healthcare and received several criticisms and calls for new administrative approaches (Morone, 1993; Spicer, 1982; Andreasson *et al.*, 2017) before switching to other administrative approaches. In general terms, the bureaucratic ritualism has been pointed out for its scarce adaptivity to new issues (Merton, 1949; Crozier, 1964), causing inefficiencies and waste of public resources (Hughes, 2003).

Then in the Eighties and Nineties the paradigm of New Public Management (Hood, 1991, 1995), emerged both in theoretical and practical ways. New Public Management, or NPM, inspired disruptive policy interventions aimed at privatization, outsourcing and deregulation of entire economic sectors (Barzelay, 2001). All over the Globe (for example in Great Britain, New Zealand, Italy) there have been implemented reforms downsizing public facilities, decentralizing responsibilities, and introducing for the public sector tools borrowed from the private for-profit sector, such as management control systems for quality and personnel.

The assumption was that the application of private-sector managerial techniques to public services would automatically lead to improvements in the efficiency and effectiveness of these services (Thatcher, 1995). Then managerialism, regionalism and quasi-markets were introduced (Le Grand & Bartlett, 1993), with particular emphasis on competition and contracting for resource allocation and service delivery, public services' disaggregation in basic units and focus on their measurement and cost management (Osborne, 2006; Ferlie et al. 1996; Ferlie & Steane, 2002).

From New Public Management to New Public Governance

The New Public Management wave was not free of critics, arguing that it was founded on an unrealistic hypothesis of individuals' rationality transferred to the public sector (Hughes, 2003) and that it emphasized managerial tools suitable for private and not for public sector, whose inner nature is the relationship between citizens and public institutions (Pollitt, 1993). In addition, the contrapositions between public and private actors was tackled as anachronistic (Mintzberg, 1996), also considering the development of the third sector. On the contrary, the mere application of business models to the management of public institutions would lead to an excessively narrow perspective, treating individuals as consumers of government's services and neglecting their roles of citizens with rights and duties, and clients with complex needs.

Other issues regarded one of the NPM's building blocks, i.e. the importance of performance measurement. The formal and a-critical adoption of performance management systems to the public sector conducted to unintended consequences (Bianchi, 2010) and to a sort of return to the bureaucratization it aimed to fight, with myopic definition of goals and indicators, lack of coordination between the political and managerial level, and between different institutions delivering public services. Apparent improvements in efficiency were not accompanied by quality advancements and value generated for the citizens (Anthony & Young, 1992).

Progressively, it became clear that *providing services is no longer a sufficient justification for State intervention funded by citizens*, that it has to be verified whether the public intervention *is achieving positive social and economic outcomes,* and that *to know whether public value is delivered requires an engagement and an exchange between the relevant stakeholders and government officials* (Stocker, 2006, p. 47). Then it was introduced a new paradigm, the New Public Governance, or New Governance (Rhodes, 1996), (also NPG in this chapter), a non-hierarchical form of government characterized by the participation of public and private actors in the design and implementation of public policies.

This approach, outcome-based and relational in nature, may produce more effective public solutions as it looks at different stakeholders' needs, opinions and values. NPG's core is that the powerful decision-making does not derive just from the formal institutional system, but from the exercise of formal and informal powers, able to create consensus about public choices through continuous interactions with the actors operating in the socio-political context (Meneguzzo, 1996).

Phases of Patients' Participation in Public Policy Making

The above discourse about public management and administration's streams of literature has highlighted how the current trend is routed into the New Public Governance, which appears suitable to explain the rationale of patient organizations' participation in the policy making. Indeed, NPG is strongly founded in cooperative policymaking: when a certain policy comes from the top, it can be either accepted or not by the stakeholders. On the contrary, involving them in the decisional process will trigger their motivation to the policy implementation, and make them open to accept the unintended consequences of certain measures.

Patient groups' involvement has been indicated as an impactful value for policy making and health research (Brett *et al.*, 2014); however, the patients' policy potential has not been fully disclosed yet, since their participation was limited to terminal steps of policy processes, with scarce attention to their perspective at early stages, such as priority setting (Liberati, 2011).

The purpose of this heading is to describe possible phases of patient-aided policy from an operational point of view. In order to address it, two reference models from literature and practice are progressively analyzed, linked and enriched to reflect patients' perspective.

The first model is the one indicated by the European Patients Forum, or EPF (Sienkiewicz & Van Lingen, 2017), which is reported in figure 1.

According to EPF, patients are involved into all the steps of policy making, the latter being considered as a funnel starting from consultation to impact, passing through policy refinement and implementation. These are the indicated steps:

1. **Consultation**: as key stakeholders of the healthcare delivery, patients can offer their perspective in stakeholder advisory groups, expert panels, European, and/or national government public consultations or institutional meetings.
2. **Policy refinement**: in a later stage, when policy was designed, patients can work on its refinements in order to improve it.
3. **Implementation**: patients can evaluate the implementation's quality of a certain policy and eventually call for new policies and recommendations.
4. **Impact**: in this stage patients are called to evaluate the policy's impact.

The EPF's model appears as a mere list of phases/stages, with no operational deepening[1]. In order to develop and detail it in a more operational way, the

Figure 1. Patient organizations' contribution to policy making process according to European Patients Forum (Sienkiewicz & Van Lingen, 2017)

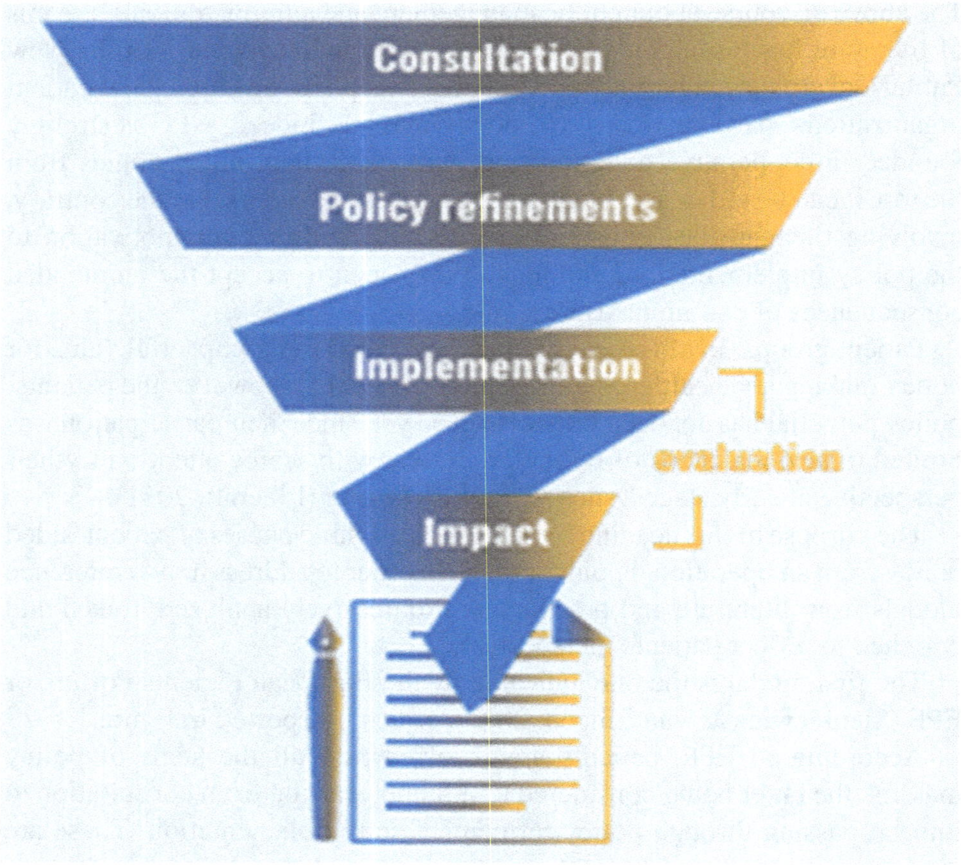

author of this chapter complements this model with the description of the 'interactive policy-making model', designed by Driessen and colleagues (Driessen *et al.*, 2001), and characterized by a more analytic and operational approach, grounded in project management and networked governance.

The authors of the second model define the interactive policy making as a *process whereby multiple parties play an active role and jointly arrive at a decision* (p. 323), in particular *government bodies collaborate with other authorities and/or private organizations to develop policy* (p. 324), and propose a management model based on six stages: exploration, initiative, common perspective, joint problem-solving, decision-making, and implementation (figure 2).

Figure 2. Steps of the interactive policy model
Adapted from: Driessen et al., 2001

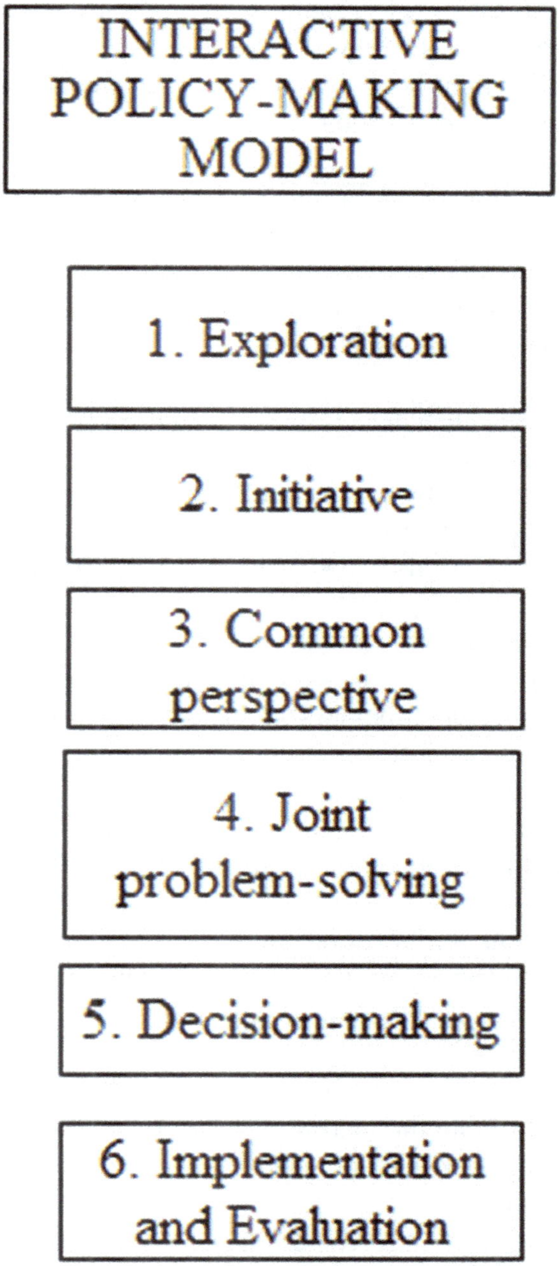

The model was built according to literature and bearing in mind the case of The Netherlands, whereas the collaborative policy making is diffuse. Notwithstanding, it still lays at a general, a-technical level; thus, in the context of the present chapter, it is believed to be adaptable to a description of the general process of patient-helped policy making. The phases of interactive policymaking are defined as follows:

1. **Exploration**: it is a preliminary phase, where the principal (the government body that will take the initiative), sketches the profile of the project in terms of the following preconditions: technical complexity, network of stakeholders potentially involved, governmental and societal context, project's timeframe, financial scope of the project (Driessen *et al.*, p. 327).
2. **Initiative**: this is the real start of the interactive policy-making project, where *the participants tell one another what they expect to gain and what they can offer* (Driessen *et al.*, 2001, p. 327).
3. **Common perspective**: this is the phase when it is determined if consensus (about problem definition and objectives) can be reached among the parties.
4. **Joint problem-solving**: in this phase it is inventoried the willingness of each party to act and to assume tasks and responsibilities during the policy implementation. At this stage it is not only important to get consensus from the working group, but also within each actor's own organization, and to *estimate how much room to maneuver will remain once the decision has been made* (Driessen *et al.*, 2001, p. 331).
5. **Decision-making**: this phase is characterized by the formalization of decisions.
6. **Implementation and evaluation**: put in action of agreements and monitoring of progresses and results, according to which *an adaptive implementation strategy can be designed* (Driessen *et al.*, 2001, p. 327).

The first phase is preliminary, is undertaken by the principal and does not consider the influence of other parties. On the other side, the initiative phase requires the interaction with other parties, because it clarifies the issues and creates in each part the commitment to be constructive in the entire process. Indeed, it is in this phase that the principal should create the stakeholders' awareness of the usefulness of the project in dealing with a common interest with policy makers and other parties. The convergence of different interests can be promoted in various ways. For example, a project group made up of patients' representatives and other social parties can prepare proposals to be discussed and/or ratified by steering committees of administrators in charge of decision-making, aided by the contribution of separated working groups in charge of specific project's aspects, due to their area of expertise and/or in representation of specific portions of society (Driessen *et al.*, 2001).

The phase of 'Common Perspective' implies to find a shared understanding of the problem. Based on the aspects set in the previous phase, this stage lets conflicts of interests emerge and tries to solve them in a creative way, i.e. forcing stakeholders to abandon their traditional view and to look for alternative ones. The problem boundaries affect the project's attitude to address the partial interests. *In that respect, one way to keep the parties at the bargaining table is to widen the scope of the problem. When the problem is broader, each one of the parties will feel that his or her own problem will get due attention in the project. Yet broadening the problem also increases its complexity* (Driessen *et al.*, 2001, p. 231).

In the 'Joint problem solving' the parties progressively agree on a certain policy option, assuming tasks and responsibilities to be accountable of in the course of implementation. Such decision needs to be supported both by the working group and by the organization and/or collectivity represented herewith, otherwise the latter could refuse to make the necessary resources available in order to achieve the objectives of the project.

The 'Decision-making' is a progressive stage where the degree of support for the decision is verified not only within the parties involved in the institutional table, but also among a wider population, through information campaigns and other tools to demonstrate the *concerted effort* (Driessen *et al.*, 2001, p. 332) also towards those parts of civil society not directly involved in the policy making.

Regarding 'Implementation', it is the formal adoption of the decided policy option, paired with the 'Evaluation' in the interactive policy-making model. It is well known in literature that policy making does not give enough space to implementation problems (Elmore, 1980; Khan, 2016). The interactive model gives an ample definition of implementation, meaning not only a practical application of what has been previously decided, but *this task also concerns whether or not these activities (and the policy objectives and strategies on which they are based) still reflect the desires and preferences of the parties most closely involved in the process* (Driessen *et al.*, 2001, p. 333).

Comparing the EPF model and the interactive policy-policy making model, the first difference lays in the number of stages in which they are articulated, respectively four and six. Notwithstanding, it is possible to track certain correspondences (represented in figure 3). The starting phase of 'Consultation' depicted in the EPF model can be considered a more synthetic way to describe the turnover between 'Initiative' and 'Common perspective' within the interactive policy-model. Or, in other terms, 'Initiative' and 'Exploration' can be seen as sub-phases of 'Consultation'. With similar logic it is possible to link 'Policy refinement' with 'Joint problem solving' and 'Decision making'.

Figure 3. Linking the European Patients Forum Model with the Interactive Policy-Making Model
(Own elaboration from: Sienkiewicz & Van Lingen, 2017, and Driessen et al., 2001)

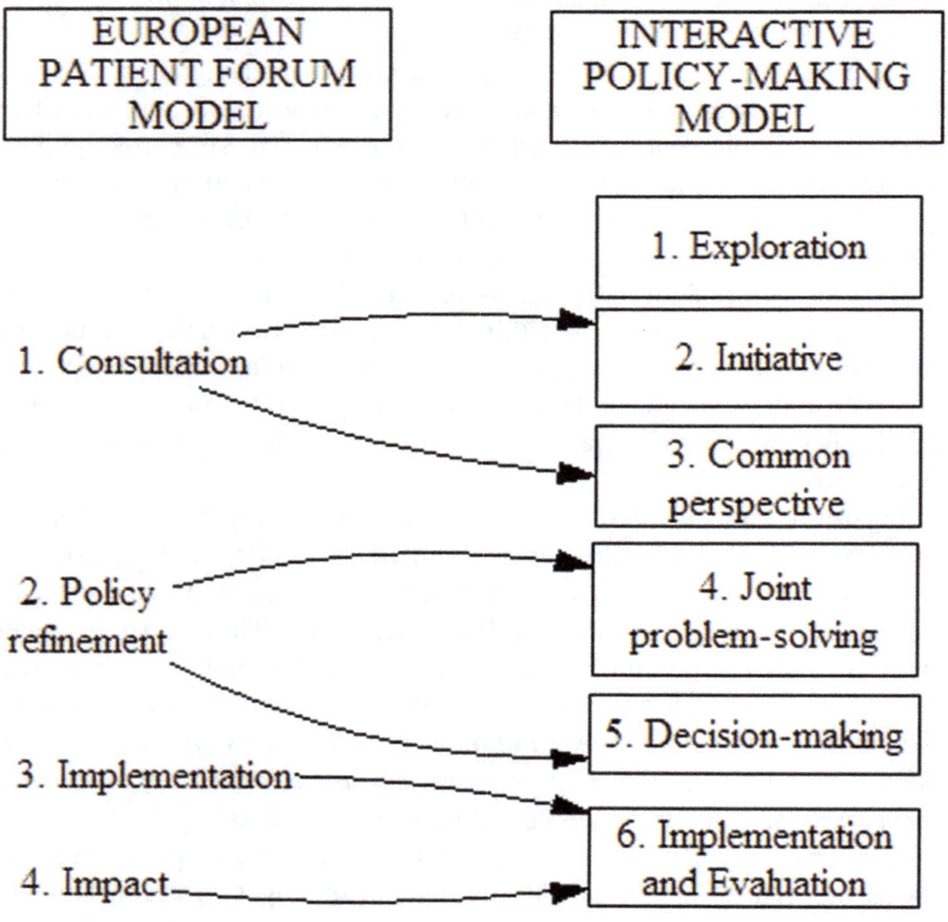

The EPF model distinguishes 'Implementation' and 'Impact', that on the contrary are expressed through a sole comprehensive phase within the interactive policy-making model. However, the biggest difference between the models is in the starting point. Indeed, while the EPF starts with 'Consultation', finding a correspondence into the interactive policy-making model, the latter starts with another stage, the 'Exploration', implying the inventory of the project's complexity, main features and risk analysis. Such element reflects the original concept of the model, i.e. public works; as well, the referral to project management issues are evident, emphasizing the role of the principal or the public body pre-seeding project ideas before taking a formal initiative. Notwithstanding, this phase, not present in the model of EPF, is equally important for the analysis of patients' contribution to the policy making process. Indeed, although patients do not directly take part in the 'Exploration' are able to sensibly affect it through the inputs provided at the point of policy implementation and evaluation, thereby directing the policy maker (i.e. the principal) in the scanning of which project to prioritize.

A Feedback View of the Interactive Policy-Making Model

The mentioned steps of the interactive policy-making model, in the authors' minds, are not to be imagined in a linear way, but as cyclical and iterative. *During the policy process feedback may be obtained from earlier phases and the policy process can also be embarked upon on several occasions* (Driessen *et al.*, 2001, p. 326). However, the authors do not represent such cyclicality and iterations. This heading aims to fill this gap and in figure 4 proposes the interactive policy-making from a feedback perspective. Even if the number of feedback loops can vary from case to case, the author of this chapter isolated some chained links, considered particularly relevant. First of all, each single step of the policy-making can be related to the 'Exploration', since an attentive policy-maker is able to take advantage of a multi-stakeholder view: the circulation of ideas and concepts, the representation of issues and priorities, the proposals of other projects, are all potentially fruitful influences coming not just from the bottom, but from the network.

Other significant loops are also represented in the right part of the scheme. On the one hand, 'Implementation' logically follows 'Decision-making' and is followed by 'Evaluation', but at the same time during the put in action of the plans it is possible the manifestation of issues not previously forecasted.

Figure 4. A feedback perspective on the interactive policy-making model

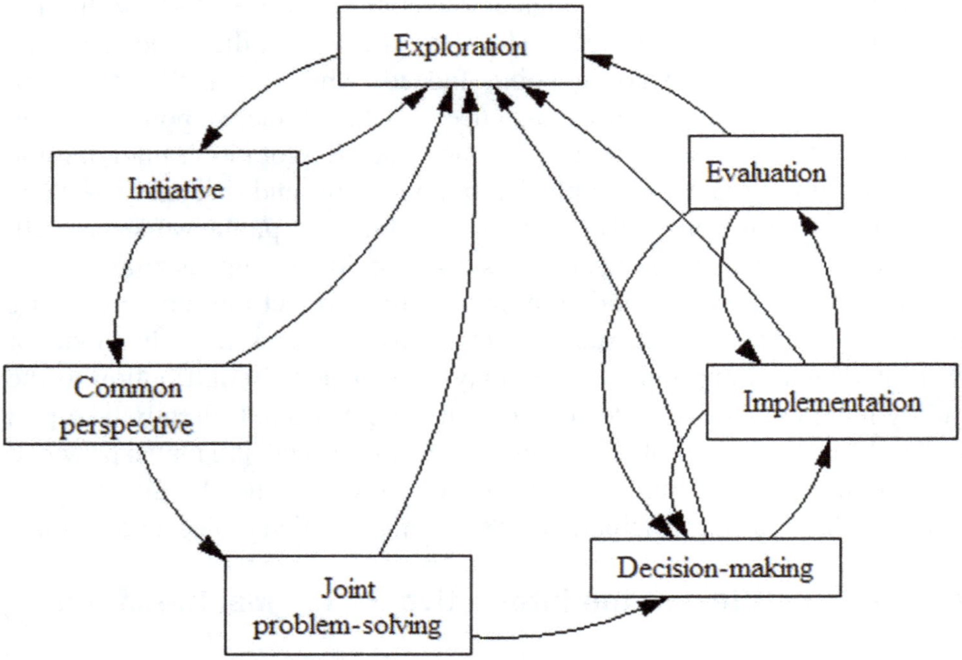

Furthermore, it is crucial to recall that the policy making is strictly connected to the process of consensus building, which must *be continuously verified in the course of the implementation process* (Driessen et al., 2001, p. 326). For these reasons, possible feedbacks can go from 'Evaluation' to 'Implementation', from 'Implementation' to 'Decision-making' or from 'Evaluation' to 'Decision-making', since new developments and insights can be used to 'Policy Refinement'. The feedback logic at the implementation stage is in line with a 'backward mapping' approach (Elmore, 1980), according to which the *specific behaviors at the lowest level of implementation is able to generate the need for a policy*, and the policy makers' perspective is integrated by considering that *other influences can affect the behavior of the people engaged in the process* (p. 604).

Table 1 analyzes some iterations taking place in the context of policy-making. They are represented as policy cycles. The major cycle, including all the stages, is the number 6, named 'Learning by experienced policies'. It can be preceded by several sub-cycles, occurring when the interaction gives rise to a

Table 1. Key interactive policy cycles

POLICY CYCLES	STAGES	DESCRIPTION
1. Policy opportunity and feasibility	Exploration → Initiative → Exploration	After a preliminary phase, the categories of stakeholders declare their expectations and the resources they made available for the project. These pieces of information can lead the principal to rethink the priorities, the project's complexity and the risks associated to the project.
2. Policy search of consensus	Exploration → Initiative →Common Perspective → Initiative	When the project reaches the step 'Common Perspective', it is possible that the interactive problem definition leads to new explorations due to: (1) other risks' detection; (2) increased complexity due to the enlargment of the projects' boundaries to compose stakeholders' interests; (3) emerging needs to include new parties into the project.
3. Policy search of solution	Exploration → Initiative →Common Perspective → Joint problem-solving → Exploration	When the project reaches the step 'Joint problem solving', it is possible that the interactive finding of solutions leads to new exploration due to the opposition to the agreed policy within the parties' own organizations.
4. Trying to put policy in action	Exploration → Initiative →Common Perspective → Joint problem-solving → Implementation → Explorations	When the project reaches the step 'Implementation', it is still possible to feed back into 'Exploration' because of possible oppositions to the agreed policy within the parties' constituencies. Moreover, too broad decisions, although easily agreed by the all parties, during implementation can be interpreted in contradictory ways and can require a general rethink of the project, or a feedback to the stage 'Joint problem-solving' (see the next policy cycle).
5. Policy refinement through implementation	Joint problem- solving →Implementation → Joint problem-solving	Too broad decisions, although easily agreed by the all parties, during implementation can be interpreted in contradictory ways (Driessen *et al.*, 2001, p. 332) and can require a feedback to the stage 'Joint problem-solving'.
6. Learning by experienced policies	Exploration → Initiative →Common Perspective → Joint problem-solving → Implementation → Evaluation → Explorations	When policy was completely implemented and evaluated, it is able to provide deep insights to the policy maker in order to guide the 'Reflection' about new policy cycles, the priorities' setting, the risks associated to certain actions, etc...
7. Implementation refinement through evaluation	Implementation → Evaluation → Implementation	During the policy implementation the continual monitoring activities could highlight implementation issues to be corrected in progress.
8. Policy refinement through evaluation	Evaluation → Joint problem-solving → Implementation → Evaluation	The progress monitoring can highlight the need to adapt the decision to the issues emerged (technical issues or lack of consensus), feeding back to the 'Joint problem solving'.

need of feedback. The latter can imply the need to go to the stage immediately backward or rather to a more radical rethink of the project's features.

In the first column each policy cycle (or sub-cycle) is numbered and named. In the second column all the policy phases been part of the cycle are listed and followed by an arrow. As obvious, the first and the last phase are always coincident, to reflect the presence of a close causal chain. In the third column a brief description of the feedback structure is provided.

FUTURE RESEARCH DIRECTIONS

This chapter examined the theoretical roots of patient engagement in policy making and the phases of decisional processes where their interventions can occur. The public management and administration's theoretical excursus remarked how New Public Governance is the opportune stream to frame patient advocacy. The model of the interactive policymaking was chosen and properly adapted to describe in more detail the patients' added value in each phase. By matching the phases reported by European Patient Forum and the ones of the interactive policy-making model, it was evaluated that the latter, although originally conceived to address policy making for public works within the Dutch context, can be adapted to patient-aided policy processes. In this regard, it is possible to see how some steps of the EPF model result in multiple steps in the second model.

Furthermore, the chapter emphasized the importance of the 'Exploration' phase, present in the interactive model and neglected in the EPF's. Since the interactive model encloses iteration and cyclicality as constituting characteristics, the chapter, keeping in mind the patients' organizations as privileged interlocutors for policy-making, proposes a further evolution of the model by providing a feedback view of the models' steps, and isolating some policy cycles that may occur before the completion of the entire process (the major loop). Future researches should deepen the analyses already conducted, by testing such framework in real policies' development, both at European and at country-specific level.

In this regard, it could be distinguished the contribution of patients' perspective in healthcare policies and in other kinds of policies connected to them (for examples social, school policies, etc…). Furthermore, it could be worth to verify the plausibility of the selected policy cycles, increasing or diminishing their number and internal composition. Finally, cross-country or cross-region analyses could also remark sensible differences in the policy models driving patients' participation, for example in some contexts the New Public Governance's perspective, privileged in this chapter, could be rather unadaptable because of the persistence of bureaucratic and New Public Management-related models. In other cases, the transition between NPM and NPG could lead to the turnover of hierarchical and cyclical processes of decision making within the same sector, for different sectors or even in dealing with differentiated cross-cutting issues.

CONCLUSION

Policy making at current times must face growingly complex issues, especially in sensitive sectors such as the healthcare one. The chapter has analyzed the roots of patients' advocacy considering public management and administration theory, as well as the patients' role in each policy making phase. In comparison to the traditional bureaucratic model and to the New Public Management, New Public Governance appears to be better suited to frame patients' advocacy. The chapter also proposes a conceptual framework by adapting the interactive policy-making model to the case of patients' advocacy. In doing so, the author enriches the analysis with a feedback view and implementation issues. The feedback view was privileged because the stages of policy processes are often presented in a linear way, even admitting (as the authors of the interactive policy-making model did) that they should be considered iterative and cyclical. This perspective has the merit to visually show how, within new governance, the politics could act to solve public issues through policy making, and the progressive and interactive completion of policy processes could stimulate at any stage new issue to deal with, new priorities to privilege, adjustments to policies previously designed.

The chapter also emphasizes the meaningfulness of implementation issues in directing policy making. On the one hand, it is recognized how policy design and implementation are sometimes conceived as two separated realities, the one unlinked to the other. This is not plausible, since implementation features are able to influence sensibly the policy outcomes. The interactive policy-making model also remarks a wider meaning of the implementation phase, more routed in the New Public Governance's way, i.e. the ability of a certain cooperative policy to still represent interests and preferences of involved parties also at the later stage of implementation. The chapter then proposes a deeper and differentiated analysis of the policy cycles and sub-cycles that could occur within a networked decisional framework. Such items complete the interactive policy-making model with relevant iterations that could stimulate reflection and adaptive policy making.

REFERENCES

Aloe, S., & De Stefano, L. (2017). *Dal Patient Engagement alla Patient Advocacy: un'evoluzione virtuosa.* Presented at Simef Italian Society of Pharmaceutic Development, Rome, Italy.

Andreasson, J., Ljungar, E., Ahistrom, L., Hermannson, J., & Delive, L. (2017). Professional Bureaucracy and Healthcare Managers' Planned Change Strategies: Governance in Swedish Healthcare. *Nordic Journal of Working Life Studies*, 8(1), 23-41.

Anthony, R. N., & Young, D. W. (1992). *Controllo di gestione per gli enti pubblici e le organizzazioni non profit.* Milano, Italy: Mc-Graw-Hill.

Balduzzi, R. (2009). Il Sistema sanitario e l'empowerment. Presentazione. *I quaderni di Monitor Agenas Agenzia Nazionale per i servizi sanitari regionali*, *6*(25), 4-6.

Barzelay, M. (2001). *The New Public Management: improving research and policy dialogue*. Berkeley, CA: University of California Press & Russell Sage Foundation.

Bianchi, C. (2010). Improving performance and fostering accountability in the Public Sector through System Dynamics modelling. From an 'external' to an 'internal' perspective. *Systems Research and Behavioral Science*, *27*(4), 361–384. doi:10.1002res.1038

Brett, J., Staniszewska, S., Mockford, C., Herron-Marx, S., Hughes, J., Tysall, C., & Suleman, R. (2014). Mapping the impact of patient and public involvement on health and social care research: A systematic review. *Health Expectations*, *17*(5), 637–650. doi:10.1111/j.1369-7625.2012.00795.x PMID:22809132

Crozier, M. (1964). *The bureaucratic phenomenon*. Chicago, IL: University of Chicago Press.

Del Fiore, L. (2016). Antonella, Patrizia e la competenza da costruire insieme. Storie di partecipazione e coinvolgimento. *Forward – Pazienti*, *3*, 2-3.

Driessen, P. P. J., Glasbergen, P., & Verdaas, C. (2001). Interactive policy-making - a model of management for public works. *European Journal of Operational Research*, *128*(2), 322–337. doi:10.1016/S0377-2217(00)00075-8

Elmore, R. F. (1980). Backward mapping: Implementation research and policy decisions. *Political Science Quarterly*, *94*(4), 601–616. doi:10.2307/2149628

EU Health Technology Assessment Network. (2014). Strategy for EU cooperation on Health Technology assessment. Brussels: EU Health Technology Assessment Network.

Ferlie, E., Ashburner, L., FitzGerald, L., & Pettigrew, A. (1996). *The New Public Management in Action*. Oxford, UK: Oxford University Press. doi:10.1093/acprof:oso/9780198289029.001.0001

Ferlie, E., & Steane, P. (2002). Changing Developments in NPM. *International Journal of Public Administration*, *25*(12), 1459–1469. doi:10.1081/PAD-120014256

Hood, C. (1991). A public management for all seasons? *Public Administration*, *69*(Spring), 3–19. doi:10.1111/j.1467-9299.1991.tb00779.x

Hood, C. (1995). Contemporary public management: A new global paradigm? *Public Policies and Administration*, *10*(2), 104–117. doi:10.1177/095207679501000208

Hughes, O. (2003). *Public management and administration. An introduction*. London, UK: MacMillan.

Khan, A. R. (2016). Policy implementation: Some aspects and issue. *Journal of Community Positive Practices*, *16*(3), 3–12.

Le Grand, J., & Bartlett, W. (1993). *Quasi-markets and social policy*. Basingstoke, UK: Macmillan Press. doi:10.1007/978-1-349-22873-7

Liberati, A. (2011). Need to realign patient-oriented and commercial and academic research. *Lancet*, 25.

Meneguzzo, M. (1996). Strategie e gestione delle reti di aziende sanitarie. Milano, Italy: Egea.

Merton, R. K. (1949). *Social theory and social structure*. New York, NY: The Free Press.

Mintzberg, H. (1996). Managing government, government management. *Harvard Business Review*, (May-June): 75–83.

Morone, J. A. (1993). The healthcare bureaucracy: Small changes, big consequences. *Journal of Health Politics, Policy and Law, 18*(3), 723–739. doi:10.1215/03616878-18-3-723 PMID:8282997

Osborne, P. S. (2006). The New Public Governance? *Public Management Review, 8*(3), 377–387. doi:10.1080/14719030600853022

Pollitt, C. (1993). *Managerialism and the public services*. Oxford, UK: Blackwell.

Rappaport, J. (1987). Terms of empowerment/exemplars of prevention: Toward a theory for community psychology. *American Journal of Community Psychology, 15*(2), 121–148. doi:10.1007/BF00919275 PMID:3604997

Rhodes, R. A. W. (1996). The New Governance: Governing without Government. *Political Studies, 44*(4), 652–667. doi:10.1111/j.1467-9248.1996.tb01747.x

Sienkiewicz, D., & Van Lingen, C. (2017). *The Added Value of Patient Organisations, Report EPF European Patients Forum Work Program*. Brussels: European Patients Forum.

Spicer, M. W. (1982). The Economics of Bureaucracy and the British National Health Service. *The Milbank Memorial Fund Quarterly. Health and Society, 60*(4), 657–672. doi:10.2307/3349695 PMID:6757787

Thatcher, M. (1995). *Downing Street Years*. London, UK: Harper Collins.

Wallerstein, N. (1992). Powerlessness, empowerment, and health: Implications for health promotion programs. *American Journal of Health Promotion, 6*(3), 197–205. doi:10.4278/0890-1171-6.3.197 PMID:10146784

Wallerstein, N. (2002). Empowerment to reduce health disparities. *Scandinavian Journal of Public Health, 30*(59_suppl), 72–77. doi:10.1177/14034948020300031201 PMID:12227969

Wallerstein, N. (2006). *What is the evidence on effectiveness of empowerment to improve health? Health Evidence Network report*. Copenhagen: WHO Regional Office for Europe.

Weber, M. (1922). *Economy and society*. Los Angeles, CA: University of California Press.

Wilson, W. (1887). The study of administration. *Political Science Quarterly*, *56*(4), 481–506. doi:10.2307/2143644

Woodal, J., Raine, G., South, J., & Warwick-Booth, L. (2010). *Empowerment and Health & Well-Being. Evidence Review*. Leeds, UK: Centre for Health Promotion Research Leeds Metropolitan University.

KEY TERMS AND DEFINITIONS

Bureaucracy: A model for public management and administration based on rationality, maintenance and legitimization of the legal power, hierarchal mechanisms, rigid definition of rights and duties, mechanical rules and procedures. In the bureaucracy there is a clear separation between the political and the administrative spheres: politicians set the goals of public institutions, while the bureaucracy gives them execution in a neutral way.

Health Technology Assessment: Evaluation of the relative assessment of a new medicine, or a treatment, or a medical device, in comparison with the others existing, in order to support decision making about fair pricings and reimbursements.

Policy: Rules to direct behaviors in specific sectors or areas of intervention, established by a government body, called policymaker, invested of the authority to set such rules. The policymakers can be supranational (e.g., the EU Parliament), national (e.g., national Parliaments and Governments), bureaucratic (e.g., departments), sectoral (e.g., utilities regulators), regional or local (e.g., regional or local councils, regional or local healthcare authorities).

Policy Evaluation: Consists on the assessment of the changes occurred due to the policy, to be measured in short, intermediate and long terms. The evaluation can take place during the policy design (before implementation) to compare the cost-benefit or cost-effectiveness of alternative policy options; during implementation, to monitor short and medium term policy outcomes; and at the end of implementation, to evaluate long term indicators of policy-driven changes (impact evaluation).

Policy Implementation: The effective execution of the policy, involving several stakeholders (both public and private) taking action to pursue policy goals. The success of a certain policy largely depends on an appropriate implementation, in terms of planned resources, skills, organizational features and risks.

Policy Options: They are the alternative policies discussed and evaluated during the policy-making process.

Project Management: Practice of initiating, planning, executing, controlling, and closing the work of a team, to achieve specific goals within project's constraints such as timing, quality requirements and budget. The core of project management is the continuous following, monitoring and governing (i.e. management) of each phase of the project. The discipline originated for the conduction of complex projects, for example for engineering, public works, software development, and so on.

New Public Governance: Form of government characterized by the participation of public and private stakeholders to the design and implementation of public policies. Such approach is non-hierarchical and according to some theorists can produce more effective public solutions because it considers needs, opinions and values of different actors.

New Public Management: Paradigm of public management and administration based on the application of private-sector's managerial techniques to public services in order to gain efficiency and effectiveness. The key policies and interventions, implemented on the New Public Management's wave in the Eighties and Nineties, included: privatizations, outsourcing, deregulation of entire sectors of the economy, public facilities' downsizing, decentralization of responsibilities, introduction of competitive logic within the public sector.

Patients' Advocacy: The participation of patients in policy making through the presence of their representatives at institutional working tables.

ENDNOTE

1 Another model from EPF, more detailed and formalized, deals with patients helping in the health technology assessment (HTA), aiming to assess the relative effectiveness of a new medicine comparing to the existing ones (Sienkiewicz & Van Lingen, 2017). Such source, used to support decisions on pricing and reimbursements (EU Health Technology Assessment Network, 2014), will not be described in this chapter, seeking instead for a general model, not routed to a specific kind of policy, like the HTA's.

Chapter 3
The Patient Added-Value to Healthcare Delivery

ABSTRACT

Patients are not considered passive recipients of the healthcare offer anymore. They can play an active role in the process of health service provision. This chapter has the scope to address the possible facets of such contribution, identifying the main areas of activity. The chapter starts with background information about service co-creation, a social and scientific paradigm born within service industry and marketing theory, recently adapted to the healthcare sector. Then the analysis continues with the description of two key spheres of patients' activities and contributions to healthcare delivery: education and research and development. It ends with conclusions and future research directions.

BACKGROUND

In the last years, advancements in service industry and in marketing theory have led to the affirmation of the value co-creation paradigm (Grönroos, 2008; Prahalad & Ramaswamy, 2000, 2004; Vargo & Lusch, 2004, 2012). The concept of value co-creation is based on the assumption that value is created by a joint effort of user/consumer and producer of a certain product or service. Such vision inverts the traditional one, based on the predominance of suppliers as value creators (Makadok & Coff, 2002; Priem, 2007). Co-creation is not limited to consumers' consultation, but it postulates the

DOI: 10.4018/978-1-7998-2653-8.ch003

pervasive integration of customers into processes of products and services' innovation (Galvagno & Dalli, 2014). In general terms, value co-creation requires a multi-stakeholder and participatory process of resource integration (Aquilani *et al.*, 2016). Yi and Gong (2013, as cited by Russo *et al.*, 2019) identify two possible co-creative behaviors: participation behaviors (search for information, information-exchange); and citizenship behaviors (provision of feedback, service promotion to other people).

A similar perspective has been recently assumed regarding the healthcare sector, aimed at overcoming the passive role of patients toward their involvement in co-creative healthcare processes (Carrubbo *et al.*, 2015). The concept of patient participation in health is not new in literature, health practice and policy making. The 1978 Alma Ata declaration of World Health Organization (WHO, 1978) stated that people's participation in the planning and implementation of their own healthcare is at the same time a right and a duty. By then, the Eighties' neoliberal policies and the *democratic deficit* observed in the 1990s, triggered all over the world a social demand for greater public accountability and the inclusion of citizens in decision-making processes (Fung & Wright, 2003, as reported by De Freitas, 2017, p. 31).

The value co-creation offers a broad paradigm in which to comprehend the key relationships between the most relevant actors of the healthcare system (e.g. doctors, nurses, patients, caregivers, administrators). On the one hand, it is well known that stakeholders within healthcare have often conflicting goals, e.g. access to services, profitability, high quality, cost containment (Porter, 2010). However, achieving high value for patients should be the overarching goal of healthcare delivery (Porter & Teisberg, 2006). Patients (like customers) can participate in the creation of health value by sharing their information, competencies and resources between each other and with health professionals (McColl-Kennedy *et al.*, 2012).

Thus, *patient becomes the most important actor in the network of value co-creation and his participation in the form of health literacy, shared decision-making, treatment control and communication with the health professionals may have several positive effects on the healthcare quality improvement* (Polese *et al.*, 2016). Despite the recognition of the importance of patients in healthcare services' co-creation, people's perception to be effectively involved is often scarce (Coulter & Jenkinson, 2005). If the program Health 2020 of the World Health Organization's (WHO, 2012) includes patient-centeredness and patients' empowerment within the priority areas for policy action, the effective adoption of co-creation in healthcare has been slow (Makhni, 2017)

Indeed, the co-creation paradigm overturns the traditional bio-medical model, based on illness treatment (Palumbo, 2016): *the 'old' concept of productivity seems to be misleading in healthcare, because it does not involve the contribution of the patient in value creation* (Nordgren, 2009). On the contrary, an informed collaborative alliance patient-physician optimizes the potential benefits of medical care (Badcott, 2005). Then, shifting away from the provider-centric model of care toward one more responsive to the needs of patients (Janamian *et al.*, 2016), involving patients in health management and improving their abilities, could contribute to healthcare sustainability, cost reduction, better health outcomes and patient satisfaction (Moretta Tartaglione *et al.*, 2018; Russo *et al.*, 2019).

The following headings will describe the healthcare co-created value through patient representative organizations. For the purpose, two main streams of intervention are addressed: (1) education; and (2) contribution to health research and development.

CONTRIBUTION THROUGH EDUCATION

The first health co-created contribution of patients through their organizations consists on the promotion of educational initiatives aimed at the dissemination of information within the healthcare and other sectors. A first distinction to be made is between the educational activities that the patient organizations entertain with people and with other organizations, both public and private. Figure 1 schematically represents the possible flows of information from and to patient organizations. As noticeable, they are located at the center, since they are at the crossroads of different sources of information: evidence-based, policy-related, condition-specific.

The relationships between patient organizations and other actors are always bi-directional: patient organizations are conceived as messengers and 'translators' between languages otherwise incompatible. By doing so, they facilitate communication dynamics between various stakeholders: doctors and patients, patients and scientific community (including applied research undertaken by private and public-private actors), patients and healthcare organizations (healthcare providers such as hospitals, clinics, community care centers), and patients and policy makers. The latter can take place through top-down and bottom-up communication mechanisms. Top-down dissemination mechanisms occur when patient organizations ease up people's understanding of policy measures; bottom-up informative movements are when patients and citizens' ideas, preferences and issues inspire policymaking. The education to other stakeholders can take place through the participation in steering committees and other institutional tables, conferences, seminars, roundtables and thematic workshops. Such meeting occasions give the opportunity to set priorities and agendas and to direct the decision making.

Furthermore, patients' organizations decode the complex information coming from organizations (policy makers, scientific community and healthcare providers) and healthcare professionals, so that they can be understood by people. The education to people can be articulated into two items: the patient community and the larger community of general population. Indeed, making complex information understandable and accessible for the patient community will build health literacy (Altin & Stock, 2015; WHO, 2013; Hoos *et al.*, 2015; Rudd *et al.*, 2004). However, the scientific and policy-related information are not to be directed just to ill people: even the civil society needs to be involved in such dissemination, in order to allow disease prevention and promotion of healthy lifestyles (Ricciardi, 2016).

On the other side, Elg and colleagues (Elg *et al.*, 2012) propose a general co-creation model where healthcare providers, in order to improve current health provision, learn from patients by collecting and analyzing their feedback. Therefore, patients' organizations could help in the collection of relevant information from the patient community and feed it to the providers, the scientific community and the policy makers.

According to the World Health Organization (WHO, 2013) health literacy is *the ability to make sound health decisions in the context of everyday life: at home, in the community, at the workplace, the healthcare system, the marketplace and the political arena*. Health literacy, allowing individuals to obtain, process, and understand basic health information and services needed to make appropriate health decisions, is recognized as a *critical enabler to engage and involve patients in their healthcare and the health of those who they care for* (Hoos *et al.*, 2015, p. 931).

In the European Patients Forum's view, health literacy *is a key determinant of health and well-being. Limited health literacy skills are associated to the underestimation of health problems (insufficient prevention and healthy lifestyles), a lack of adherence to treatment and/or self-management of chronic conditions, the subsequent aggravation of health inequities, more frequent hospitalizations and emergency care utilizations. Better health literacy can support prevention and healthy lifestyles, prevent medical mistakes, and improve the effectiveness of health systems thanks to active patients and citizens* (Sienkiewicz & Van Lingen, 2017, p. 13). Thus, high-quality of care

Figure 1. Flow of information from and to patients' organizations

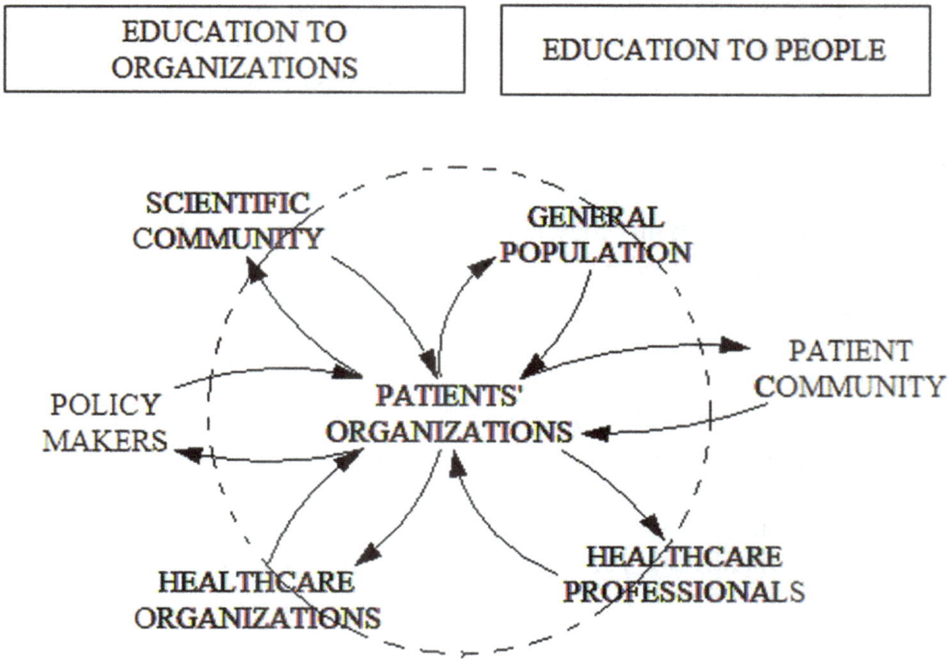

requires *an improvement of patient capabilities to navigate through the layers of healthcare systems that become more and more complex and demanding* (Paasche Orlow *et al*., 2006, as cited by Altin & Stock, 2015, p.184).

The pervasive dissemination of healthcare-related knowledge (about epidemiology, typologies of treatments and quality of life) requires the involvement of several stakeholders, like health professionals, advocacy groups, researchers, European institutions and national governments, digital and non-digital media, and vulnerable groups such as chronically ill, deprived and elderly populations, mostly affected by limited health literacy (World Health Organization, 2013). Health literacy is also required for patients' involvement into health Research & Development processes (addressed in the next heading of the chapter).

In this regard, patients' organizations can make scientific information comprehensible for patients and civil communities. This implies: (1) to translate from a language to another documents and guidelines, (2) to adapt them to context-specific issues, (3) to collaborate in the writing of health information materials for patients, enriching them with non-medical information still important for patients' life (e.g. healthy diets, social inclusion's features, reimbursements), (4) to educate people on their equal treatment rights (both to accessible and quality healthcare and to other public services).

These figures assume a crucial role at current times of digital transformation: on the one hand the patients are potentially informed due to the plenty of health-related information on the internet (Greene *et al.*, 2011; Lee *et al.*, 2015; Ahmed *et al.*, 2017), in particular about treatment options or self-care. On the other side, patients may not be able to discern credible sources of information and/or to make sense of it. In this case, the educational value of patient organisations helps patients to make the best possible use of such opportunities.

Regarding the potential participation in clinical trials, even though researchers explain to patients the meaning of such experiments, legal and professional jargons are not easily understandable. Then patients' organizations often shed light on this complexity and make it more accessible. In addition, when several clinical trials are available for the same disease at the same time, patient organizations can support the best suited choice.

CONTRIBUTION TO HEALTH RESEARCH & DEVELOPMENT

Patients' interventions to enhance healthcare delivery can also take place in the sphere of health research. Several studies have emphasized how empowering patients and let them participate in the shaping of healthcare and health research can improve the quality of these processes (among the others, Mockford *et al.*, 2012; O'Mara-Eves *et al.*, 2013). Substantially, patients' organizations are involved in data collection and advisory: such activities connote an overlapping, grey zone, between health research and policy making spheres, especially as far as priority setting and budget allocations. In this heading the health research co-creative processes are distinguished into two main categories: health research, and pharmaceutical Research & Development.

Patients and Health Research

Patients' inclusion in health research means *new ways of science co-creation* (Sienkiewicz & Van Lingen, 2017, p. 15), where patients' inputs lay at all stages of the research process, including the development of user-focused research objectives and research questions, more appropriate recruitment strategies, consumer-focused interpretation of data and enhanced implementation and user-friendly dissemination of study results (Brett *et al.*, 2012).

The added value of patient organizations is in bringing patient experience on certain diseases, identifying priorities and assessing the impact of different treatments. In this respect, disease-specific organizations, collecting empirical data through questionnaires and maintaining patient registries and biobanks, enrich *the political and practical narrative within the health research area through contextual background, wider community development, and empowerment* (Sienkiewicz & Van Lingen, 2017, p. 15). Nevertheless, for the evidence-based healthcare, seen by governments as a solution to rising healthcare costs, poor quality, and safety concerns, the determination of a patient's treatment requires to balance scientific evidence, practitioner judgment, and patient's experiences and preferences (USA National Working Group on Evidence-Based Healthcare, 2008). Figure 2 represents the possible movements of information and inputs coming from patients within the health research continuum. The scheme was built following the recommendations on the policy report 'The Role of the Patient/Consumer in Establishing a Dynamic Clinical Research Continuum: Models of Patient/Consumer Inclusion', by the USA National Working Group on Evidence-Based Healthcare (2008).

In the scheme above, patients start to contribute - together with other stakeholders - to health research in the stage of 'Research Prioritization', helping researchers to identify unanswered questions or research gaps. This can happen by let them participate in preclinical research focus-groups that identify new research targets. Patients and their organizations can also propose and develop research studies. In the next phase, 'Research Study Development', patients can be involved in defining key questions and research methodologies, as well as consumer-focused clinical or quality of life endpoints. The patients' perspective can be fruitful also in the stage of

Figure 2. Patients' contribution to evidence-based healthcare

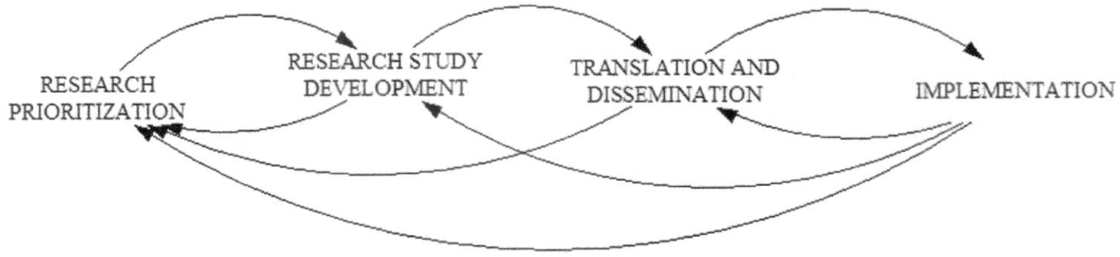

'Translation and Dissemination', through the test of key findings derived from evidence development, and focus groups contributing to many possible areas: translation of informative materials to a wider audience, formulation of communication strategies (channels, tools, and networks to disseminate research effectively and efficiently), development of educational products for targeted audiences. Patient inputs can also be useful to identify health literacy needs, areas for further research, barriers to research implementation, i.e. obstacles to the incorporation of research information into patient practice and clinical interactions. In the 'Implementation' stage patients and representative organizations can be part of the advisory panels and stakeholder dialogue with decision-makers (public and private) to identify key lessons from evidence, inform coverage and reimbursement policies, track patient health outcomes, identify any access-to-care issues, new targets for policy changes, map intended and unintended consequences, monitor impacts based on patient-focused outcomes (USA National Working Group on Evidence-Based Healthcare, 2008).

Finally, it is easy to notice that the process is conceived as a feedback loop, since patient inputs at later stages can be used to start other researches, defining and prioritizing post-market research needs within government regulatory bodies and promoting the development of new studies. The digital transformation favored the patient-led research by mean of new ways of data collection, with people sharing their health data online to help each other and track progresses, by using smartphones, digital health records, online portals (Tozzi & Gesualdo, 2017). These possibilities gave rise to the production of new kinds of data, enhancing the ongoing empowerment of patients, not mere passive recipients of medical prescriptions and advices, but *actively measuring and interacting, within communities where they have a powerful voice in the direction and conduct of learning* (Sienkiewicz & Van Lingen, 2017, p. 16). Policy makers recognize big data as important sources to conduct researches (for example European Commission, 2016). Then patients' organizations play the twofold role of (1) promoting the interest of patients in sharing their health data; (2) promoting good governance and regulation of data access and use in order to protect patients' privacy (Sienkiewicz & Van Lingen, 2017, p. 16).

Another application of patient involvement in health research is the partnership in peer-reviewed scientific publications. For example, the British Medical Journal in 2014 adopted a strategy of patients' inclusion into the research process (British Medical Journal, 2014). Indeed, the journal considers partnering with patients and their networks as a necessary step to promote quality and sustainable health research and systems. Patients and advocates are members of the journal's editorial board and are involved in discussions and decision making. The authors wishing to submit research papers to the journal must document if and how they have co-created them with patients through various steps of research process (formulation of research questions, establishment of outcome measures, studies' design and implementation, dissemination of results). In any case, each submitted work (even the ones not carried out with patients' collaboration) after a preliminary evaluation (done by editors), is reviewed both by academic and patient referees (chosen within a database of patients, patients' advocates, and caregivers).

Patients and Pharmaceutical Research and Development

In the pharmaceutical Research & Development, the role of patients has recently shifted from the mere, traditional participation in clinical trials to the inclusion at early stages of Research & Development of medicines and medical treatments devices. Even the pharmaceutical industry has recognized the importance to focus unmet medical needs of patients since the beginning of the development process, which otherwise can lead to wrong priorities, wrong decisions on research design, and potentially costly late-stage failures (Hoos *et al.*, 2015, p. 929). In this context, patient organizations facilitate patients and community's involvement in the development and review of clinical trial protocols, and contribute to the branch of health technology assessment (HTA), used to support decisions on pricing and reimbursements (EU Health Technology Assessment Network, 2014).

Health Technology Assessment is defined as *the systematic evaluation of properties, effects, and/or impacts of health technology* (Integlia & Mazzoni, 2017, p. 11). The tremendous technological progress has led to advances in healthcare delivery and patient outcomes, which in turn made healthcare costs to increase. Then HTA is primarily utilised to provide inputs to decision making, in assessing intended and unintended consequences (safety, efficacy, effectiveness, cost, and cost-effectiveness, ethical and legal implications) of new health technologies (medicines, treatments, devices), both in absolute terms and comparing them with competing ones. Then it requires a multidisciplinary approach studying medical, social, ethical, and economic implications of development, diffusion, and use of health technologies.

As far as patient involvement in R&D is concerned, according to Hoos and colleagues (Hoos *et al.*, 2015, p. 930), like in other industries, product development should begin with a clear understanding of the needs of the end-users, namely the patients; but in spite of the medicines' intrinsic purpose to improve patients' lives and to provide more effective healthcare, current inclusion practices during development and lifecycle management are fragmentary and mostly confined to post-launch or late-stage clinical development. The same authors summarise perceived risks and barriers to patient involvement (table 1).

A more comprehensive approach of patients' involvement into the pharmaceutical R&D is represented in the roadmap in figure 3, adapted from a work of Geissler and colleagues (Geissler *et al.*, 2017). A similar map is also reported in the guidelines for patients' involvement in HTA (Hunter *et al.*, 2018), developed by the European Patient Forum within the project EUPATI (European Patients' Academy). The latter distinguishes three different definitions of patients (Hunter *et al.*, 2018, p. 3): (a) Individual Patients: persons experiencing the co-existence with the disease. They do not necessary have technical knowledge in Research & Development or regulatory processes, since their role is to contribute with their subjective disease and treatments' experience; (b) Patient Organization Representatives:

Table 1. Perceived risks and barriers to patient involvement (adapted from Hoos et al., 2015, p. 935)

Critical areas	Perceived risks and barriers to patient involvement
Education and training	• Educational needs of stakeholders, including scientific literacy • Lack of a common understanding of what patient involvement entails • Need for training and guidance on effective patient involvement
Communication	• Need for effective communication with appropriate phrasing that is understood by all stakeholders and that reflects the diversity of the patient population • No agreed on a comprehensive definition of patient
Perceptions and cultural barriers	• Perception that patient involvement is driven primarily by regulatory concerns • Phenomenon of tokenism, where patients are involved but their inputs are not truly heard and acted upon • Perception of patient engagement as a 'soft' science • Perception of engagement with patients as risky • Need for a cultural shift to accept the importance of patient engagement • Need to establish an environment of mutual trust and respect, openness and reciprocity
Evidence	• Lack of robust evidence for the benefits and value of patient involvement
Structure, support, and resources	• Structure, support, and resources • Logistics and support required to ensure wide patient representation • Availability of resources to develop and implement patient involvement initiatives
Legal and regulatory	• Impact of legal and regulatory restrictions on the industry's and other stakeholders' communication with patients

they represent and express the collective views of a patient organization on a specific issue or disease area; (c) Patient Experts: differ to the individual patients because beside their disease-specific expertise, they have technical knowledge in R&D and/or regulatory affairs through training or experience.

The chart presents the possible ways of patients' involvement along four key stages of medicine lifecycle of R&D: (1) Research Priority Setting, (2) Research Design and Planning, (3) Research Conduct and Operations, (4) Dissemination, Communication, and Post-Approval. Patient-aided activities are different depending on the patients' level of expertise: on the top of the figure, there are the ones involving expert patients in the required disease area, on the bottom part there are activities that can be carried out by non-expert patients in the specific area of disease. In comparison with the original model, in the one represented herewith, expert and non-expert patients' contributions have been numbered for better clarity in showing which R&D's stage each activity belongs to.

In the research upstream level, i.e. 'Priority Setting', only highly expert patients can play a relevant role, verifying the alignment between research priorities and patient needs, defining patient-relevant added value and patient-relevant outcomes, and ensuring R&D processes focusing on *areas of patient care that require improvement as defined by patients themselves* (Geissler *et al.*, 2017, p.2).

In the second stage, 'Research Design and Planning', both expert and non-expert patients can have a significant weight. On the upper part of the

Figure 3. Patients' involvement in Research and Development of medicines (adapted from Geissler et al., 2017, p.5)

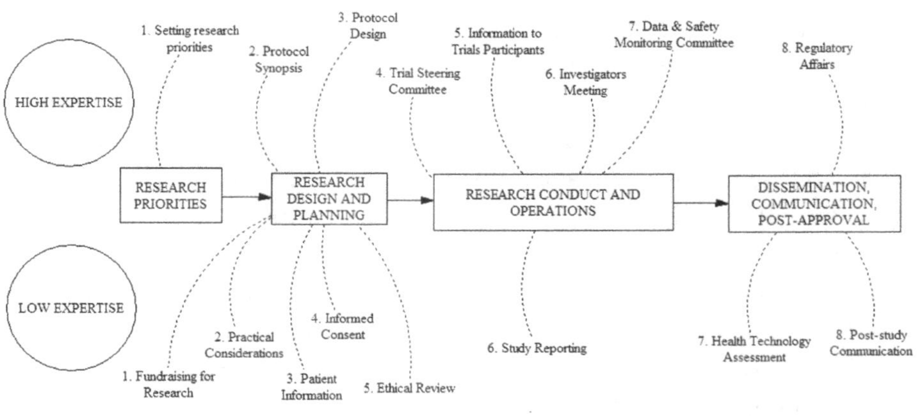

roadmap, two activities are ascribable to expert patients: protocol synopsis and protocol design. In these contexts, patient inputs can help for example in identifying relevant endpoints of the cure, acceptable risks versus potential benefits, the relevant target population; defining the criteria of inclusion and exclusion to the clinical trial; selecting relevant patient-centred outcomes measures such as quality of life (Bellini & Kubler, 2018; Mc Lean *et al.*, 2019). The possible contributions of non-expert patients in this stage are several: (1) fundraising, in particular for new research topics; (2) identification of practical considerations (travel expenses, support for family members, etc…); (3) identification of relevant information able to affect the willingness to take part to the trial, for example data protection. In this case, useful are patients' personal advices about quality content, and clear and readable informative materials to approach potential participants, such as leaflets and (4) informed consent forms; (5) ethical review, where patients' inclusion helps to assess if the research wishes to bring meaningful outcomes for the target population and if it is managed so as to take into consideration needs and preferences of participants, to find an equilibrium in the trade-off between need of personalized care and sensitive data collection.

In the third stage, i.e. 'Research Conduct and Operations', patient representatives firstly can take part to trial steering committees and to investigator meetings. In such working tables the patients' perspective can help in detecting ongoing challenges and opportunities, promoting changes in the protocol, to be properly communicated to the participants emphasizing reasons and effects on patients' safety. Later, patient representatives can work in monitoring committees for data & safety, where their view can help to evaluate the impact of study results on real patients, facilitating the assessment of side effects. Furthermore, the non-expert patients, through representative organizations, can make study reports, communicating the achievement of clinical trials' milestone results to the wider patient community, thereby improving patient access to trials.

Finally, in the fourth stage ('Dissemination, Communication, and Post-Approval') expert patients can play a role in regulatory affairs (marketing authorizations, development and revision of results' reports, package leaflets) by involving their representatives into advisory groups within international and national agencies and authorities. The European Medicines Agency, or EMA (2016), involves three categories of expert patients and representatives to different kinds of activities: (1) patients as individual experts are assigned to product-related activities (scientific advices and protocol assistance procedures, scientific advisory expert groups, scientific committees' consultations, review of documents); (2) patients representing their organization (i.e. the organizations they belong because of their health status) are involved in non-product related activities such as EMA consultations and workshops; (3) patients representing the general world of patient organizations contribute with more strategic activities, like the participation in the management boards and to the scientific committees.

On the other side, non-expert patients are involved into HTA and post-study communication activities. Health Technology Assessment requires to evaluate whether previously identified patient priorities and patient-relevant outcomes have been appropriately addressed, whilst among the post-study communication strategies there is the development of synopses of results for the wider patient and professional communities.

FUTURE RESEARCH DIRECTIONS

The chapter made a general review of patients' participation in the provision of healthcare, addressing the topics of value co-creation through education and research, and reporting selected literature's contents. Future research steps could shed light into specific aspects of such mechanisms, like the ethical conflicts that could occur in protocol designs, the risk that patients involved in research can influence each other, the resource management for patients' inclusion into researches, the time for training and education of both patients and researchers (Brett *et al.*, 2012). Other works could deal with barriers to patients' participation in Health Technology Assessment, due to discouraging attitudes of HTA organizations, considering HTA as a scientific process whereas patient input is seen as anecdotal or biased (Hunter *et al.*, 2018, p. 9). Next researches should also focus the relationships between patient organizations and other stakeholders, putting attention to public-private partnerships and making international comparisons. The distinction made in the chapter between contribution through education and contribution to health Research & Development was done for explanatory purposes. However, there are many links between these two categories of patients' contribution, reinforcing each other in virtuous dynamic mechanisms, to be better addressed in future works.

CONCLUSION

This chapter remarked how co-creative mechanisms can take place in the healthcare sector by treating patients as customers. Two core roles of patient representative organizations have been described: education and research. Regarding the contribution through education, patients' organizations were framed as central actors interfacing and decoding different actors and languages, whilst the contribution to the research process was analysed distinguishing health and pharmaceutical research and identifying possible steps and applications.

REFERENCES

Ahmed, S., Haines-Saah, R. J., Afzal, A. R., Tam-Tham, H., Al Mamun, M., Hemmelgarn, B. R., & Turin, T. C. (2017). User-driven conversations about dialysis through Facebook: A qualitative thematic analysis. *Nephrology (Carlton, Vic.)*, *22*(4), 301–307. doi:10.1111/nep.12780 PMID:27003709

Altin, S. V., & Stock, S. (2015). Impact of health literacy, accessibility and coordination of care on patient's satisfaction with primary care in Germany. *BMC Family Practice*, *16*(1), 148–154. doi:10.118612875-015-0372-0 PMID:26492959

Aquilani, B., Silvestri, C., & Ruggieri, A. (2016). Sustainability, TQM and Value Co-Creation Processes: The Role of Critical Success Factors. *Sustainability*, *8*(10), 995–1017. doi:10.3390u8100995

Badcott, D. (2005). The expert patient: Valid recognition or false hope? *Medicine, Health Care, and Philosophy*, *8*(2), 173–178. doi:10.100711019-005-2275-7 PMID:16215797

Bellini, M., & Kubler, A. (2018). Health Literacy and Patient-Reported Outcomes. In *Optimizing Health Literacy for Improved Clinical Practices* (pp. 109–123). Hershey, PA: IGI Global. doi:10.4018/978-1-5225-4074-8.ch007

Berkman, N. D., Sheridan, S. L., Donahue, K. E., Halpern, D. J., & Crotty, K. (2011). Low Health Literacy and Health Outcomes: An Updated Systematic Review. *Annals of Internal Medicine*, *155*(2), 97–107. doi:10.7326/0003-4819-155-2-201107190-00005 PMID:21768583

Brett, J., Staniszewska, S., Mockford, C., Herron-Marx, S., Hughes, J., Tysall, C., & Suleman, L. (2012). Mapping the impact of patient and public involvement on health and social care research: A systematic review. *Health Expectations*, *17*(5), 637–650. doi:10.1111/j.1369-7625.2012.00795.x PMID:22809132

British Medical Journal. (2014). *Patient and public partnership*. Retrieved August 20, 2019, from https://www.bmj.com/campaign/patient-partnership

Carrubbo, L., Bruni, R., Cavacece, Y., & Moretta Tartaglione, A. (2015). Service System Platforms to Improve Value Co-Creation: Insights for Translational Medicine. In Service Dominant Logic, Network and Systems Theory and Service Science: Integrating Three Perspectives for a New Service Agenda. Napoli, Italy: Giannini Editore.

Coulter, A., & Jenkinson, C. (2005). European patients' views on the responsiveness of health systems and healthcare providers. *European Journal of Public Health*, *15*(4), 355–360. doi:10.1093/eurpub/cki004 PMID:15975955

Davis, M. A., Anthony, D. L., & Pauls, S. D. (2015). Seeking and receiving social support on Facebook for surgery. *Social Science & Medicine*, *131*, 40–47. doi:10.1016/j.socscimed.2015.02.038 PMID:25753284

De Freitas, C. (2017). Editorial Public and patient participation in health policy, care and research. *Porto Biomedical Journal*, *2*(2), 31–32. doi:10.1016/j.pbj.2017.01.001

Elg, M., Engström, J., Witell, L., & Poksinska, B. (2012). Co-creation and learning in health-care service development. *Journal of Service Management*, *23*(3), 328–343. doi:10.1108/09564231211248435

EU Health Technology Assessment Network. (2014). Strategy for EU cooperation on Health Technology assessment. Brussels: EU Health Technology Assessment Network.

European Commission. (2016). *Study on Big Data in Public Health, Telemedicine and Healthcare*. EU Publications Office.

European Medicines Agency. (2016). *European Medicines Agency's interaction with patients, consumers, healthcare professionals and their organizations - Annual report 2015 (EMA/727872/2015)*. Amsterdam: Stakeholders and Communication Division.

Fung, A., & Wright, E. O. (2003). *Deepening democracy. Institutional democracy in empowered participatory governance*. London, UK: Verso.

Galvagno, M., & Dalli, D. (2014). Theory of value co-creation: A systematic literature review. *Journal of Service Theory and Practice*, *24*(6), 643–683.

Geissler, J., Ryll, B., Leto di Priolo, S., & Uhlenhopp, M. (2017). Improving Patient Involvement in Medicines Research and Development: A Practical Roadmap. *Therapeutic Innovation & Regulatory Science*, *51*(5), 1–8. doi:10.1177/2168479017706405 PMID:30231692

Greene, J. A., Choudhry, N. K., Kilabuk, E., & Shrank, W. H. (2011). Online social networking by patients with diabetes: A qualitative evaluation of communication with Facebook. *Journal of General Internal Medicine*, *26*(3), 287–292. doi:10.100711606-010-1526-3 PMID:20945113

Grönroos, C. (2008). Service Logic Revisited: Who Creates Value? And Who Co-Creates? *European Business Review*, *20*(4), 298–314. doi:10.1108/09555340810886585

Hoos, A., Anderson, J., Boutin, M., Dewulf, L., Geissler, J., Johnston, G., ... Tougas, G. (2015). Partnering With Patients in the Development and Lifecycle of Medicines: A Call for Action. *Therapeutic Innovation & Regulatory Science*, *49*(6), 929–939. doi:10.1177/2168479015580384 PMID:26539338

Hunter, A., Facey, K., Thomas, V., Haerry, D., Warner, K., Klingmann, I., ... See, W. (2018). EUPATI Guidance for Patient Involvement in Medicines Research and Development: Health Technology Assessment. *Frontiers in Medicine*, *5*(231), 1–10. PMID:30238004

Integlia, D., & Mazzoni, E. (2017). Health Technology Assessment in Europe. State of arts and future scenarios. Rome, Italy: Icom Institute for Competitiveness.

Janamian, T., Crossland, L., & Wells, L. (2016). On the road to value co-creation in healthcare: The role of consumers in defining the destination, planning the journey and sharing the drive. *The Medical Journal of Australia*, *204*(7), 12–14.

Lee, J. L., Choudhry, N. K., Wu, A. W., Matlin, O., Troyen, A. B., & Shrank, W. H. (2016). Patient Use of Email, Facebook, and Physician Websites to Communicate with Physicians: A National Online Survey of Retail Pharmacy Users. *Journal of General Internal Medicine*, *31*(1), 45–51. doi:10.100711606-015-3374-7 PMID:26105675

Makadok, R., & Coff, R. (2002). The theory of value and the value of theory: Breaking new ground versus reinventing the wheel. *Academy of Management Review*, *27*, 10–13.

Makhni, S. (2017). From the Editor: Co-Creation in Health Systems Design. AMA Journal of Ethics, 19(11), 1070-1072.

Mc Lean, K. A., Drake, T. M., Sgrò, A., Camilleri-Brennan, J., Knight, S. R., Ots, R., ... Harrison, E. M. (2019). The effect of liver transplantation on patient-centred outcomes: A propensity-scorematched analysis. *Transplant International*, *32*(8), 808–819. PMID:30793373

McColl-Kennedy, J. R., Vargo, S. L., Dagger, T. S., Sweeney, J. C., & van Kasteren, Y. (2012). Healthcare customer value cocreation practice styles. *Journal of Service Research*, *15*(4), 370–389. doi:10.1177/1094670512442806

Mockford, C., Staniszewska, S., Griffiths, F., & Herron-Marx, S. (2012). The impact of patient and public involvement on UK NHS healthcare: A systematic review. *International Journal for Quality in Health Care*, *24*(1), 28–38. doi:10.1093/intqhc/mzr066 PMID:22109631

Moretta Tartaglione, A., Cavacece, Y., Cassia, F., & Russo, G. (2018). The excellence of patient-centered healthcare: Investigating the links between empowerment, cocreation and satisfaction. *The TQM Journal*, *30*(2), 153–167. doi:10.1108/TQM-11-2017-0138

Nordgren, L. (2009). Value creation in healthcare services - developing service productivity: Experiences from Sweden. *International Journal of Public Sector Management*, *22*(2), 114–127. doi:10.1108/09513550910934529

O'Mara-Eves, A., Brunton, G., McDaid, D., Oliver, S., Kavanagh, J., Jamal, F., . . . Thomas, J. (2013). Community engagement to reduce inequalities in health: a systematic review, meta-analysis and economic analysis. In Public Health Research (Vol. 1.4). Southampton, UK: NIHR Journals Library.

OECD. (2013). *Skills outlook 2013. First results from the survey of adult skills*. Paris: OECD Publishing.

Paasche Orlow, M. K., Schillinger, D., Greene, S. M., & Wagner, E. H. (2006). How healthcare systems can begin to address the challenge of limited literacy. *Journal of General Internal Medicine*, *21*(8), 884–887. doi:10.1111/j.1525-1497.2006.00544.x PMID:16881952

Paasche-Orlow, M. K., Schillinger, D., Greene, S. M., & Wagner, E. H. (2006). How healthcare systems can begin to address the challenge of limited literacy. *Journal of General Internal Medicine*, *21*(8), 884–887. doi:10.1111/j.1525-1497.2006.00544.x PMID:16881952

Palumbo, R. (2016). Contextualizing co-production of healthcare: A systematic literature review. *International Journal of Public Sector Management*, *29*(1), 72–90. doi:10.1108/IJPSM-07-2015-0125

Polese, F., Moretta Tartaglione, A., & Cavacece, Y. (2016). *Patient empowerment for healthcare service quality improvements: a value co-creation view*. Paper presented at the 19th Toulon-Verona International Conference, Huelva, Spain.

Porter, M. E. (2010). What is value in healthcare? *The New England Journal of Medicine*, *363*(26), 2477–2481. doi:10.1056/NEJMp1011024 PMID:21142528

Porter, M. E., & Teisberg, E. O. (2006). *Redefining healthcare: creating value-based competition on results*. Boston, MA: Harvard Business School Press.

Prahalad, C. K., & Ramaswamy, V. (2000). Co-opting customer competence. *Harvard Business Review*, *78*(1), 79–87.

Prahalad, C. K., & Ramaswamy, V. (2004). *The future of competition: co-creating unique value with customers*. Boston, MA: Harvard Business School Press.

Priem, R. L. (2007). A consumer perspective on value creation. *Academy of Management Review*, *32*(1), 219–235. doi:10.5465/amr.2007.23464055

Ricciardi, W. (2016). Health literacy: un diritto dei cittadini, un dovere delle istituzioni. *Forward – Pazienti*, *3*, 3.

Rudd, R., Kirsch, I., & Yamamoto, K. (2004). *Literacy and Health in America: A Policy Information Center Report*. Princeton, NJ: Educational Testing Service.

Russo, G., Moretta Tartaglione, A., & Cavacece, Y. (2019). Empowering Patients to Co-Create a Sustainable Healthcare Value. *Sustainability*, *11*(5), 1315–1334. doi:10.3390u11051315

Sienkiewicz, D., & Van Lingen, C. (2017). *The Added Value of Patient Organisations, Report EPF European Patients Forum Work Program*. Brussels: European Patients Forum.

USA National Working Group on Evidence-Based Healthcare. (2008). *The Role of the Patient/Consumer in Establishing a Dynamic Clinical Research Continuum: Models of Patient/Consumer Inclusion*. Retrieved July 18, 2019, from http://www.evidencebasedhealthcare.org/images/download/W.G.PatientConsumerBklt2%288-6%29.pdf

Vargo, S. L., & Lusch, R. F. (2004). Evolving to a New Dominant Logic for Marketing. *Journal of Marketing*, *68*(1), 1–17. doi:10.1509/jmkg.68.1.1.24036

Vargo, S. L., & Lusch, R. F. (2012). The Nature and Understanding of Value: A Service- Dominant Logic Perspective. *Review of Marketing Research*, *9*, 1–12. doi:10.1108/S1548-6435(2012)0000009005

World Health Organization. (1978). *Alma-Ata Primary healthcare, Health for all series, n. 1*. Geneva: WHO Regional Office for Europe.

World Health Organization. (2012). *Policy Framework and Strategy Document*. Geneva, CH: WHO Regional Office for Europe.

World Health Organization. (2013). *Health literacy: the solid facts*. Copenhagen, DK: WHO Regional Office for Europe.

Yi, Y., & Gong, T. (2013). Customer value co-creation behavior: Scale development and validation. *Journal of Business Research*, *66*(9), 1279–1284. doi:10.1016/j.jbusres.2012.02.026

ADDITIONAL READING

Bernhardt, J. M., Brownfield, E. D., & Parker, R. (2005). Understanding Health Literacy in J. G. Schwartzberg, Van Geest, J. B. & Wang C. C. (eds.), Understanding Health Literacy: Implications for Medicine and Public Health. Chicago, IL: American Medical Association.

Gauvin, F. P., Abelson, J., Giacomini, M., Eyles, J., & Lavis, J. N. (2010). It all depends: Conceptualizing public involvement in the context of health technology assessment agencies. *Social Science & Medicine*, *70*(10), 1518–1526. doi:10.1016/j.socscimed.2010.01.036 PMID:20207061

KEY TERMS AND DEFINITIONS

European Medicines Agency (EMA): Decentralized agency of the European Union responsible for the scientific evaluation, supervision and safety monitoring of medicines in the EU. It is a networking organization whose activities (carried out by the scientific committees) involve thousands of experts across Europe.

Research Design: A detailed methodological plan guiding the entire research. It is a framework of methods and techniques chosen by the researchers to address the research questions. Thus, the focus is on how the research is going to be conducted and contains explanations about data collection methods, measurement and analysis. The design has to be neutral (not biased), reliable (if research is repeated, similar results are expected); valid (the measuring tools chosen for the research have to lead to relevant results for the specific ongoing research); and generalizable (the research results should be extended from the sample to a wider population). The research design can be quantitative or qualitative, depending on whether statistical conclusions are required for the study. It can also be descriptive (only describing the issue under research); experimental (aiming to state causal relationships between independent and dependent variables); correlational (to establish if there exists a relation between two variables, with no statement of what causes what else); diagnostic (deep analysis of the causal tissue of a certain topic); explanatory (where the researcher provides personal ideas and thoughts about a certain theme).

Research Synopsis: The plan of a certain research protocol, providing the rationale, the main objectives, and the methods for data collection. Standard synopses are usually organized in the following headings: title (to be short, clear and self-explanatory), that can be enriched by a more descriptive sub-title; abstract, which is a brief summary (150-200 words) of the stated problem, research goals, theories and methods; introduction (providing background information about the addressed problem); detailed literature review about the research problem; objectives of the study (in turn based on the literature review); hypotheses (prediction of the outcomes of the study in terms of relations between variables); limitations, i.e. specific aspect of the problem not addressed by the study; methodology and methods suitable to achieve the objectives of the study, where the researchers choose a comprehensive methodology (experiments, surveys, models, case studies) within which it is possible to use different methods (qualitative and quantitative) for data collection and analysis; results (analyses of data, organized in tables and graphs); discussion (connection of the results to the objectives); conclusion (about research contribution and recommendations for future studies); literature references.

Value Co-Creation: Paradigm based on the assumption that value is created by a joint effort of user/consumer and producer of a certain product or service. Such vision inverts the traditional one, based on the predominance of suppliers as value creators, and postulates a multi-stakeholder participatory process of resource integration. Value co-creation can also be applied to the healthcare sector, to switch the patient from a mere recipient of professionals' directives toward a more active and creative role.

Chapter 4
Knowledge and Skills to Lead Effective Patient Organizations

ABSTRACT

The potential role of patients' organizations in healthcare, in order to be effective, needs to be sustained by appropriate knowledge and skills. The chapter has the scope to review the key requirements for the management of such organizations. After a background introduction about added value of patient capacity building, it proposes the 'antenna skill framework', a visual and practical illustration summarizing the necessary knowledge and skills for patient organizations' management. A generic patient organization is represented as an antenna progressively picking up many kinds of knowledge and skills: about the institutional framework, disease-related, technical, and managerial. Particular attention is devoted to management and administration, proposing a business model canvas tailored to patient organizations. In conclusion, the insightful tools proposed in the chapter can foster policymakers, universities, and other educational operators to conceive suitable training programs to form capable patient managers.

BACKGROUND

The contribution of patient organizations to health policies and healthcare R&D, as well as the educational role of patients' organizations to disseminate information from patients to other stakeholders (policy-makers, health authorities, mass media, scientific community, professional community)

DOI: 10.4018/978-1-7998-2653-8.ch004

and vice-versa, require for these entities a strong attitude to internal capacity building and to strengthen their organizations and governance structures (Sienkiewicz & Van Lingen, 2017). Ideally, patients' organizations should assume the connotation of learning organizations, 'places' where people collectively learn how to learn, continually developing new patterns of thinking and the capacity to achieve desired results (Senge, 1990). Such organizations, whereas 'organizational learning' takes place (Rebelo & Gomes, 2011; Tsang, 1997) are also innovative and performing (Power & Waddell, 2004; Watkins & Marsick, 1993; 1999; Robinson *et al.*, 1997), because they are able to adapt to environmental changes (Armstrong & Foley, 2003). According to Watkins and Marsick (1993), seven dimensions connote learning organizations: continuous learning, dialogue and inquiry, team learning, embedded system, system connections, empowerment and leadership. More recently Marquadt (2011) identified five sub-systems in a learning organization: organization, learning, people, knowledge management, and technology. Each of them complements and is dynamically interrelated with the others: consequently, a scarce development in one (or more) of these subsystems has a compromising effect on the entire organizational system.

The above literature highlights how a holistic and systemic approach is needed to manage effective organizations. The scope of the present chapter is to propose a general framework summarizing the necessary knowledge and skills for patient organizations' management. In order to address this aim, the core categories of desired knowledge and skills are identified according to managerial and policy literature. Afterwards, the categories are 'exploded' into more specific areas and put together in the 'antenna skill framework', a visual and practical framework summarizing the necessary knowledge and skills for patient organizations' management. The notion of skills used in this chapter consists on *the ability to apply knowledge and use know-how to complete tasks and solve problems* (https://ec.europa.eu/esco/portal/escopedia/Skill). In some cases, the term 'skills' is paired with 'knowledge', to remark that some practical and technical applications require important achievements and advancements in one's cognitive sphere (about basic or specialist concepts and ideas) to be practiced systematically. When the term 'skills' is used alone, it is because the practical/technical component is prevalent in comparison with the - still present - epistemological one (for example in the case of communication skills).

PROPOSING A FRAMEWORK OF RELEVANT KNOWLEDGE AND SKILLS

In this section it is proposed the 'antenna skill framework', a representation summarizing the necessary knowledge and skills for the management of patient organizations. The building of this tool has followed two main steps: in a first phase, there were identified four macro-categories of desired skills (or knowledge and skills); in a second moment, each category previously identified was split into more specific areas to be developed by patients' organizations.

The macro-categories of skills and knowledge, represented in figure 1, were included according to relevant citing literature and training and educational needs expressed by patients' organizations. According to the European Patients Forum, one of the key internal challenge for patient organizations is the organizational professionalization and know-how (Sienkiewicz & Van Lingen, 2017, p. 20). Indeed, these entities often miss skills of strategic planning, fundraising, communication. These deficiencies can be ascribable to lack of earmarked funding, understaffing, underdeveloped knowledge base, lack of technical and bureaucratic language used by EU institutions and national authorities. Such figure finds confirmation in an Italian survey about leadership in 193 patients' organizations (ALTEMS, 2018). This source shows how patient organizations' leadership skills present strengths and weaknesses. On the one hand, the role of patients' representation in policy making together with other health stakeholders is mainly based on a knowledge matured directly on the field and never formalized. On the other side, despite satisfying levels of leadership's motivation, empathy and capacity of networking, areas of improvement are technical and management-related, for example financial planning, fundraising and human resource management.

The macro-categories identified are the following:

1. **Health Related Knowledge and Skills**: The inclusion of this category is justified by the embeddedness of patients' organizations into the healthcare sector.
2. **Management and Administration Knowledge and Skills**: This category encloses technical and managerial skills.
3. **Technology Related Skills**: Includes both information and communication technology and social media management.

4. **Soft Skills**: These skills are transversal, i.e. usable also in other fields of life.

Each macro-category was furtherly exploded in more specific areas, and logically framed into the 'antenna skill framework' (figure 2). The unit of analysis is a generic patients' organization, from which all the selected areas of knowledge and skills radiate. The name of this visual structure was chosen reminding the design and functions of an antenna, able to receive and to transmit signals. Indeed, organizations are open systems entertaining many exchanges (material, financial, informative) with the reference environment (physical and socio-economic); thus, the practice of any skill within organizations cannot be separated from a continual reference to the reference system. All the skills must be cultivated synergistically for the survival of the organization and the success of the initiatives carried out, while learning processes can take place both through formal educational paths and/or by doing day-by-day operations. In this regard, the proposed representation is also intended to be a sort of insightful agenda to inspire training programs to form capable patient organizations' managers. For a better intelligibility of the scheme, circular labels are placed next to the areas of knowledge and skills belonging to the original groups.

Looking at the figure 2 from the top, it is possible to notice a sequence of items in rectangular boxes of decreasing size. These are the key areas of health-related knowledge and skills, whereas the funnel-like representation is justified because each item should 'contain' the one below and 'be contained' by the one above. The last step of the cascade is the 'disease specific knowledge', i.e. the nearest - and easiest to access - item for the patients' organization. The more you descend along the chain, the smaller the width of the information and the greater the depth, with specific focus on patients' issues. The chain can also be started to read with a bottom-up approach: the disease-related knowledge is progressively enriched by knowledge and capacity building about the steps of health research and the principles of patient empowerment and advocacy, as well as about healthcare organizations and healthcare systems in general terms.

If one means to use the scheme in figure 2 as a critical reminder for patient educational and training activities, the first approach appears more suitable as a start in the context of formal learning, because it goes from general, ample spectrum definitions and concepts, to more specific and focused ones. However, creating a strong basis of healthcare related knowledge and skills is not enough to lead successful patients' organizations. The latter requires

Figure 1. Desired knowledge and skills' categories for patients' organizations

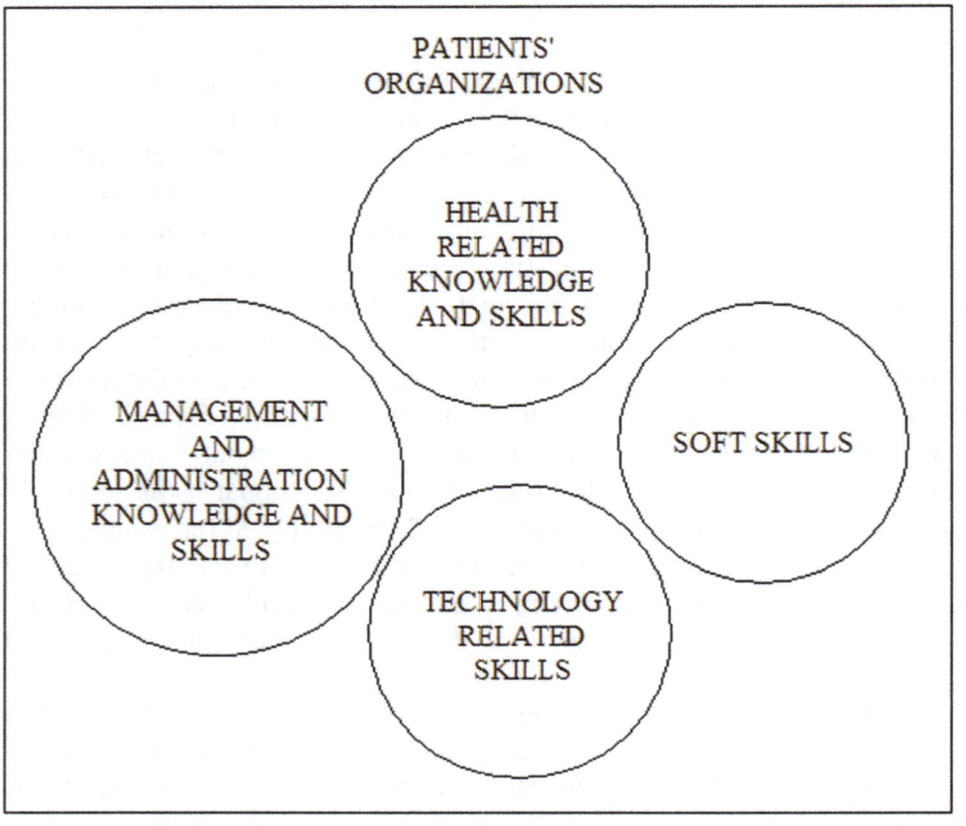

to develop other kinds of technical, managerial, technological and soft skills, which radiate from the center of the figure. In the next headings of the chapter, a description of each constituent part of the framework will be provided. The examination does not claim to be exhaustive as it just deals with the core aspects linked to the challenges of today's patient organizations.

HEALTHCARE RELATED KNOWLEDGE AND SKILLS

This section of the 'antenna skill framework' provide the core contents of four types of knowledge and skills:

Figure 2. General framework of knowledge and skills for effective patient organizations' management

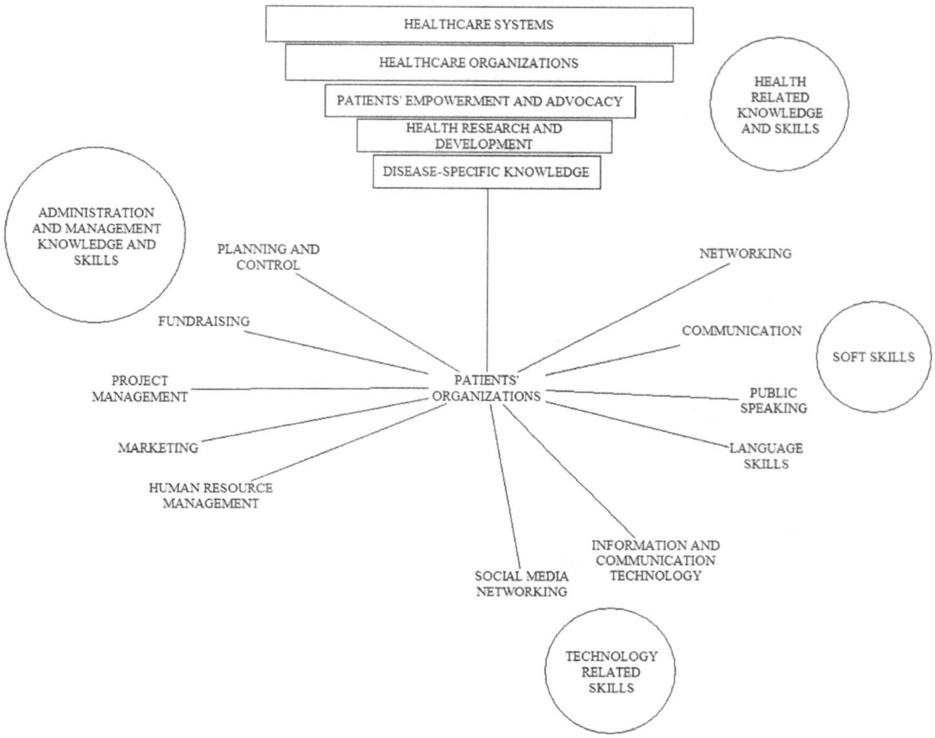

1. **Healthcare Systems**: goals of the healthcare systems, providers, financial resources, typologies of funding systems (general taxation, national health insurance, voluntary or private health insurance, out-of-pockets payments, donations to charities); institutional frameworks; key stakeholders and their relationships; health regulations.
2. **Healthcare Organizations**: typologies of healthcare providers, private and public, functioning and relationships with other stakeholders, economic and financial sustainability, phases and processes of healthcare delivery, management and administration, criteria of resource allocation.
3. **Patient Empowerment and Advocacy**: patient-centered healthcare (Cooper *et al.*, 2016; Selby & Lipstein, 2014), possible contributions of patients' involvement in health policy making and in the healthcare delivery (Brett *et al.*, 2014).

4. **Health Research and Development**: specific focus on the contributions of patients' involvement in health research and development, typologies of research, distinction between activities for expert patients and for those not receiving specific training and education on health research phases and expert patients (Hunter *et al.*, 2018).
5. **Disease-Specific Knowledge**: patients experience their own conditions so that they are privileged interlocutors to talk about it. Especially regarding chronic illnesses, they coexist with the pathologic condition all the life long, and they possess higher expertise than any other involved stakeholder about it (Rathert *et al.*, 2011, 2013; Bovaird, 2007). The concept of disease-specific knowledge is meant in a wide sense, to cover not only the medical aspects of diagnosis, treatment and follow-up, but also the procedural knowledge behind these milestones, for example the bureaucratic requirements to book an outpatient visit, the steps for treatments, the financial requirements to carry out the cures, and so forth. Such knowledge is implicit in patients but must be formalized within patients' organizations (Del Fiore, 2016; Weinberger, 2011) in order to be properly communicated to people needing information, e.g. the ones suspecting to be ill or the general population for prevention's scopes.

MANAGEMENT AND ADMINISTRATION KNOWLEDGE AND SKILLS

Patients' organizations are NGOs, thus being part of the third sector. They do not belong neither to governments nor to the for-profit sector (Salamon & Anheier, 1996) and form a sub-set of organizations within civil society that are international, regional, national or locally based (Lambell *et al.*, 2008). According to Salamon and Anheier (1996) five basic features distinguish NGOs from other kinds of organizations:

1. They are organized: it means that they are institutionalized to some extent. The institutional characteristic can be ascribable to a legal charter of incorporation or through a persistent internal organizational structure, with enduring goals and recognized boundaries between members and non-members. Therefore, temporary gatherings of people with no real structure or organizational identity are not to be included into the NGOs.

2. They are private: they are not part of government's apparatus, which in turn does not exercise any authority on them. This does not mean that they cannot receive government support, but that they have an institutional identity separate from that of the state.
3. They are self-governing: they are equipped to control their own activities to a significant extent through internal governance procedures.
4. They do not distribute profits and reinvest them into activities related to the mission of the organization. Although nonprofit organizations are not primarily driven by commercial goals and considerations, this does not mean that management models and techniques typical of the private business sector may not apply to NGOs, with proper adaptations.
5. They are voluntary: the voluntarism has two different - coexisting - meanings: (1) in order to be included in the nonprofit sector, the organization must engage volunteers in its management (board participation) or operations through the use of voluntary resources (time of staff volunteering or financial donations); (2) the second is that the membership has not to be compulsory, i.e. volunteering and donations have not to be required or established by law.

A Business Model Canvas Tailored to Patients' Organizations

In line with Osterwalder & Pigneur's thoughts (2010), although NGOs are not enclosed into the for-profit sector, they can have a business model, i.e. a representation of how they create, deliver, and capture value, with the word 'business' not used as a descriptor (p. 264). These authors have developed a general framework, the 'business model canvas', a tool for describing, analyzing, and designing business models. It is an immediate representation of how strategies can *be implemented through organizational structures, processes and systems*. The canvas of for-profit organizations is made of nine building blocks (covering the business areas of customers, offer, infrastructure, and financial viability):

1. **Customer Segments**: Groups of people or organizations an enterprise aims to reach and serve. They can be grouped in segments with homogeneous needs, behaviors or other relevant attributes.

2. **Value Propositions**: An aggregation of benefits that the company can offer to customers, thus consisting on the main reason why customers prefer one company in comparison to the others.
3. **Channels**: This building block describes how the company communicates with and reaches its customer segments to deliver a value proposition.
4. **Customer Relationships**: This is a building block illustrating the types of relationships a company establishes or wants to establish with specific customer segments.
5. **Revenue Streams**: The cash a company generates from each customer segment, from which costs must be subtracted to obtain earnings.
6. **Key Resources**: Necessary assets to make a business model work, since they allow the company to create and offer a value proposition. There can be physical, financial, intellectual, or human key-resources, that can be owned or leased by the company or acquired from key partners.
7. **Key Activities**: These are the most important activities the company undertakes on a regular basis in order to make its business model work and to create and offer a value proposition.
8. **Key Partnerships**: This section presents the network of suppliers and partners helping to make the business model work.
9. **Cost Structure**: This block is made of all the necessary costs to operate a business model, descending from key resources, activities and partnerships.

This framework can be used both for describing as-is and to-be business models. When dealing with *beyond-profit business models*, Osterwalder & Pigneur (2010, p. 264) distinguish two cases, admitting the possibility of blended business models incorporating the characteristics of them both:

- **Third-Party Funded Enterprise Models**: in this business model the recipients of products or services are not the payers. Indeed, a third party (for example philanthropies, charities, governmental bodies), pays the organization to fulfill a mission, which may be of social, ecological, or public service nature. Such organizations' business models disclose the risk of incentives' misalignments: the third-party financer becomes the main customer, so that *the incentive to create value for donors may be stronger than the incentive to create value for recipients*;
- **Triple Bottom Line Business Models**: Characterize the organizations with a strong ecological and/or social mission. The 'triple bottom line' means to account not only for financial performance, but also for

environmental and social ones, so that the business model canvas needs to have inserted two more building blocks: (a) social and environmental costs (negative impacts), and (b) social and environmental revenues (positive impacts).

The Osterwalder & Pigneur's framework can be adapted to a patients' organization (table 1), by considering a blended business model incorporating elements of the third-party business models and the triple bottom line business models. Indeed, as in the third-party funded enterprises models, among the core sources of funds for this kind of organizations, there are donations and grants, often coming from governmental bodies or the pharmaceutical industry. The patients' organizations receiving funds from the industry take the risk of conflicts of interests, able to undermine the credibility of the entire organization in front of the patients and the civil community. This is not likely to happen in the case of public grants because of the 'physiological social mission' of States and supra-national governments bodies. On the other side, as in the triple bottom line business models, patients' organizations have a strong social mission, so that beside financial costs and revenues, also social and environmental costs need to be taken in proper consideration.

The peculiarity (and complexity) of the business model canvas tailored to patients' organizations is the fact that several actors can play multiple roles within the same value proposition: for example, the patients' community is both a customer segment and a key partner; whilst the policy maker and the pharmaceutical industry at the same time are key partners, provide key financial resources and thereby represent customer segments. So far, the value proposition is to defend patients' interests through patients' support, education, empowerment, engagement, involvement and advocacy. In order to deliver it, key activities are peer support, participation in policy making and R&D, educational and training support: several key partners reflect such orientation.

Key resources to carry out the necessary activities for value propositions are mainly financial (public grants, funds from the pharmaceutical industry, donations, participation fees) and human (voluntary work, healthcare and disease-related expertise, management and administration skills, soft skills, technology skills), that can be owned by the patients' organizations or progressively acquired from key partners.

The customer segments are patients' community, pharmaceutical industry and policy makers. With them the relationships must be collaborative and

Table 1. Business model canvas of a patients' organization

<table>
<tr>
<td rowspan="2">KEY PARTNERS
- Patient community.
- Other patients' organizations for the same or for other diseases, at the same or at other territorial levels (local, regional, national, international).
- Healthcare providers.
- Scientific community.
- Pharmaceutical industry.
- Agencies for Health Technology Assessment.
- Healthcare professionals.
- Policy makers.</td>
<td>KEY ACTIVITIES
- Peer support to their members, to the patient community and to the civil society.
- Educational activities to several actors, included feedback to health providers and professionals.
- Training activities to the patients.
- Participation in health R&D.
- Participation in policy making.</td>
<td rowspan="2">VALUE PROPOSITION
To defend patients' interests through patients' support, education, empowerment, engagement, involvement and advocacy.</td>
<td>CUSTOMER RELATIONSHIPS
- Collaborative relationships with patients' community, healthcare providers, pharmaceutical industry, policy makers.
- Transparent relationships with specific funding actors (e.g. the pharmaceutical industry) to mitigate potential conflicts of interests.</td>
<td rowspan="2">CUSTOMER SEGMENTS
Patients' community.
Pharmaceutical industry.
Policy makers.</td>
</tr>
<tr>
<td>KEY RESOURCES
- Public grants.
- Funds from the pharmaceutical industry.
- Donations.
- Participation Fees.
- Voluntary work.
- Healthcare and disease-related expertise.
- Management and Administration knowledge and skills.
- Soft skills.
- Technology skills.</td>
<td>CHANNELS
Dissemination of knowledge and information through:
- traditional and social media marketing campaigns;
- pamphlets and other informative materials;
- events such as conferences, seminars and workshop.
Capacity building through programs and courses.</td>
</tr>
<tr>
<td colspan="3">COST STRUCTURE
- Office rent.
- Volunteers' compensation/refund.
- Purchase of computers and office equipment and materials.
- Purchase of printing services and merchandise goods.
- Purchase of traditional or social media marketing services.</td>
<td colspan="2">REVENUE STREAMS
- Public grants.
- Funds from the pharmaceutical industry.
- Donations.
- Participation Fees.
- Charity merchandises and sales, spontaneous offers.</td>
</tr>
<tr>
<td colspan="3">SOCIAL AND ENVIRONMENTAL COSTS
- Possible conflicts of interests.
- Delay in policy decision-making.</td>
<td colspan="2">SOCIAL AND ENVIRONMENTAL REVENUES
- Universal access to healthcare.
- Improvement of healthcare quality.
- Diffusion of healthy lifestyles.
- Effective policy making, social cohesion.</td>
</tr>
</table>

transparent, especially with specific funding actors (e.g. the pharmaceutical industry) to mitigate potential conflicts of interests.

The channels of communication with customer segments are traditional and new media campaigns, conferences, seminars, workshops, capacity building programs and courses. The costs are for renting offices, compensating volunteers for their time, providing the office with computers, equipment and materials, and purchasing printing and merchandising goods for dissemination initiatives. Also marketing services are likely to be purchased whenever the corresponding skills are not internally developed. The revenue streams are three types: (1) coming from third parties (public grants, funds from the pharmaceutical industry, donations) normally representing the most relevant sources, (2) deriving from the voluntary membership enrolment (participation or association fees), and (3) coming from charitable initiatives (charity merchandises and sales, spontaneous offers).

The last layer of the business model canvas reflects the social mission of patients' organizations, whose positive impacts (social and environmental revenues) are improvements of accessibility and quality of healthcare, diffusion of healthy lifestyles, effective policy making and thereby social cohesion. On the other side, the negative impacts (social and environmental costs) are ascribable to potential delays related to the interactive policy making (Driessen *et al.*, 2016), and not managed conflicts of interests.

In the European context, the European Patients Forum (EPF) laments poor grants for the systematic involvement of patients and their organizations. The reduction of public health and health research's budgets has caused some patients' organizations to accept private sources of funding from pharmaceutical industry (for operational activities or for specific projects). The latter potentially brings conflicts of interests, undermining the credibility of patients' organizations. Then EPF proposes a two level mechanism: European Union should establish core grants, whilst member States should explore, in cooperation with patients' organizations and private sector's partners, *innovative and ethical options for funding patient groups that will enable them to function and maintain their independence from industry and from the government* (European Patients Forum, 2016). Poor understanding of how patients' organizations work with industry partners and how they prevent conflicts of interest also causes public trust to reduce. In order to mitigate such issues, many patients' organizations have developed clear rules for transparency, ethical conduct and engagement's codes of practice, also in collaboration with pharmaceutical industries (see for example European Federation for Pharmaceutical Industries and Associations, 2011).

Required Managerial and Administration Knowledge and Skills

The business model above basically contains, among the key resources to value proposition, the same knowledge and skills of the 'antenna skill framework': healthcare related (in particular, disease-specific), management and administration, soft skills and technology skills.

Particular attention was devoted to managerial and administration skills, since their lacking has been reported by the European Patients Forum (Sienkiewicz & Van Lingen, 2017, p. 20), focusing the missing of strategic planning, fundraising, communication, ascribable to shortage of funding, understaffing, underdeveloped knowledge base, linguistic lacks. The ALTEMS survey (2018) on leadership of patients' organizations also identifies issues in passing the bell from one leader to another, due to scarcity of professionally trained profiles, with prevalence of informal learning processes and problematic areas in the financial planning, fundraising and human resource management. Indeed, it was remarked by Lewis (2001) that NGOs, as primarily informal and person-driven, may have the tendency to underestimate the importance of the organizational aspect, sometimes perceived as distractive from their actual work. Referring to developmental NGOs, three overlapping roles can be played: (a) mobilization of resources, to provide goods and services to people or to other stakeholders, in order to improve overall service quality, as part of the NGO's own project or that of a government or donor agency; (b) a 'catalyst role' of inspiring changes in other actors through social capital, empowerment-based approaches, lobbying and advocacy work, innovation and influence to policy processes; (c) a partnering role with government, donors and the private sector, which implies the capacity to build meaningful relationships. The latter requires the NGOs' ability to manage complex relationships, especially with the industry, and the need to be accountable to several stakeholders.

The same author in a later work (Lewis, 2003) proposes a framework for the management of NGOs. Premising that third sector's organizations are distinct from businesses because they do not make a profit, and from government agencies since their authority is not derived from political process, He believes that NGOs' management is not a separate field, but a composite item, made of a mix of multiple sources of management ideas from other fields, characterized by an 'improvisational nature'. Then NGOs' management needs to take insights from the following fields:

- Generic business management theory, especially as far as strategic planning (Fowler, 1997) is concerned. This is because NGOs are organizations like any other and should give priority to well established management figures (accounting, recruiting, training etc…), drawn from the business world;
- Third sector management: the NGOs, part of the third sector, may face challenges such as the appropriate use of volunteers and the strategies for fund-raising, and then require specialized approaches for which generic management may not apply. These structural characteristics call for specific models and concepts, not to be a-critically transferred from other sectors (Billis, 1993);
- Public sector management: because NGOs are often engaged with service delivery to citizens and public policies.

However, the management models and tools from the above fields do not have to be applied straightforward, but *it is an improvisational process of innovation and adaptation by NGOs that makes the flexible use of management ideas and tools succeed or fail* (Lewis, 2003, p. 339). For Korten (1987) such organizations, created to meet people's immediate needs, over the time develop more sophisticated agendas and need structural changes. Such discourses apply suitably to patients' organizations, that according to the European Patients Forum, lack organizational professionalization, and, among the others, miss skills of strategic planning and fundraising (Sienkiewicz & Van Lingen, 2017, p. 20). For them, in figure 2, left sided, five areas of knowledge and skills to be developed were specified:

1. **Planning and Control**: The management must set in advance objectives (strategic, tactic, operational) for the organization and how to achieve them. At the same time, there must be controlling procedures to verify (both during implementation and afterwards) the level of fulfillment of objectives, in order to analyze the causal tissue of gaps and undertake corrective actions. Precondition to effective organizational Planning and Control is the presence of effective accounting systems and the implementation of performance measurement systems, absent or just anecdotal within patients' organizations (Sienkiewicz & Van Lingen, 2017, p. 19). Indeed, performance-based incentives (monetary or non-monetary) are worthy stimuli to employees' commitment to the organizational mission, goals, objectives, and values (Batti, 2014, p. 93).

2. **Fundraising**: The activity of requiring financial support to public and private actors. It constitutes the principal source of revenues for non-profit organizations. Fundraising activities cannot be improvised and must be properly managed and controlled. After developing the goals of the organizations and the activities to be carried out to achieve them, a fundraising plan needs to be developed to establish the desired amounts of money to raise, the funding sources, and the related fundraising initiatives that the organization will undertake. Such plan is likely to be modified in pace with new inputs, issues and opportunities emerging from the operational activities. The plan also contains a timeline for all the activities to be carried out, and an esteem of the costs associated to them, e.g. to create and run websites, to organize events, to compensate staff specifically dedicated to fundraising. The plan must be evaluated all the yearlong (for example, every two or three months), adopting criteria such as money collected, number of new donors, average donation amount per donor and per category of donors, new contacts developed through the events organized. The assessing of such results will help to understand critical success factors and to underline possible paths of improvement (for further details about fundraising, see https://www.thebalancesmb.com/fundraising-plan-new-nonprofit-2502113).
3. **Project Management**: A project is the planning to achieve a specific objective, which involves a series of activities and tasks that consume resources and require the respect of certain quality standards and time constraints. The project management is the process of ensuring the achievement of the project objectives by applying a collection of tools and techniques, making the best use of the existing organizational structures and resources, without compromising the routine operations of the company (Munns & Bjeirmi, 1996). Project management skills are relevant for patients' organizations, since they are often project-oriented or involved in initiatives having projects' core characteristics, i.e. unique ventures characterized by explicit goals and quality requirements, with limited timeframes and important budget limitations.
4. **Marketing**: Several researches emphasize the importance of market orientation for the non-profit sector (Kotler, 1979; 1982; Kara *et al.*, 2004; Padanyi & Gainer, 2004; Sargeant *et al.*, 2002) in achieving organizational missions. The patients' organizations can need to communicate messages to other stakeholders about their scopes, activities, events. Thus, it is important that marketing skills are developed within the organizations or acquired from outward. In order to develop appropriate marketing

campaigns, it is crucial to identify target audience groups to eventually direct differentiated messages, to propose effective messages, and to integrate several instruments within the marketing strategy (sponsorships, advertisement, social media marketing, podcasts, etc...).

5. **Human Resource Management:** Human resource management is the part of management concerned with people at work and their relationships within the organization (Stanley, & Albin, 2013). The attention to it by NGOs is normally relatively scarce, whilst successful NGOs are those that recognize the significance of the human factor for organizational success (Batti, 2014). The project orientation of many patients' organizations can mean *low priority for investing in nurturing human resource capacities and staff retention measures due to the short-term nature of the projects* (p. 90). In addition, when the size of organization is small, no units of human resource management are created. The function is informally handled by project managers or staff members, with possible creation of confusion about roles and responsibilities. Like any other NGOs, because of financial shortages patients' organizations do not have the possibility to provide benefits to motivate human resources. Indeed, the compensations to working people largely depends on donor funds and public grants, thereby undermining staff morale and organizational performances (p. 91). For these reasons, for patients' organizations is crucial to develop, within their Planning and Control activities, human resource management plans able to link human resource capacity and organizational goals, and incentivizing mechanisms other than the financial ones (p. 92). For example, capacity through courses and training paths, as well as creating a strong and conducive organizational culture, can be motivating for staff members to commit to the organizational goals. Finally, it is of capital importance to develop management and leadership's succession plans. This requires identifying which employees have the potential to take up leading positions and to develop programs to build specific competencies (p. 93).

SOFT SKILLS

The 'antenna skill framework' in figure 2 includes a section dedicated to some soft skills that need to be enforced in patients' organizations, represented on the right area of the scheme. Soft skills have been recognised as *essentials for NGOs positions and play an important role in the implementation of daily activities in NGOs' jobs* (Hajjaj & Mandysova, 2017). Regarding the patients' organizations, the relevant items are: networking, communication, public speaking and language skills.

Networking implies the creation of direct or indirect links between nodes, allowing to develop strategic competitive advantage (De Man, 2004). In the business context, the managers' ability to create connections is considered conducive to highly performative organizations (see, among the others, Kay, 2004; and Boe, 1994). Some people have an innate propensity towards networking, others need to acquire it through experience and educational paths. For this reason, it is recommended that educational systems, managers and policymakers focus on networking as a part of management training (De Klerk, 2010).

Networking activities (and the related skills) are valuable for NGOs to enhance their performance and to create synergies with key actors at different institutional levels, avoiding dispersion of energies and resources, and enforcing their impacts on societies. The patient organizations' networking skills can be analyzed together with the disease-specific knowledge by considering the framework in figure 2. This was developed by Moreira (2014) to define epistemic identity of patients' organizations as function of the relationship between knowledge activities and network integration.

Moreira starts his analysis by studying the hystory case of an Alzheimer patients' organisation with regard to the contribution to health technology

Figure 3. Epistemic identity of patients' organizations as function of the relationship between knowledge activities and network integration. Source: (Moreira, 2014, p. 3356)

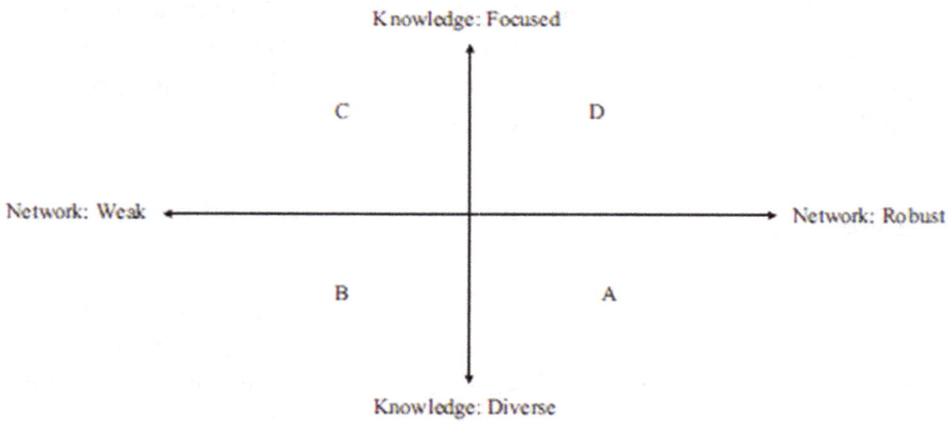

assessment, chosen because it *underpins much of the knowledge and evidence that is brought to bear in healthcare decision making* (p. 3350). Nevertheless, for such health conditions, the involvement in HTA's research is historically associated with a strong participation in expert and policy networks at national and global levels. According to the study, the dynamic relationship between the knowledge produced by this organization and the networks of expertise and policy mobilized, shaped the organization's identity as knowledge producer according to three stages (Moreira, 2014).

In the first stage, the organization set its mission in provision of patient and caregivers' mutual support and of information about the illness, to members and the public. Then the organizational knowledge was focused on experiential knowledge and put emphasis on volunteer membership, links with clinicians and public support. In the second stage, the organization re-shaped its knowledge identity from experiential to hybrid, i.e. *as a combination of experiential, clinical and scientific knowledge in an attempt to redraw its relationship with volunteers and to expand its field of activism into HTA* (p. 3352). In the third phase, the organization expanded its network of organizations for a wider production of evidence and for a unique contribution in policy making (Moreira, 2014).

For Moreira this case study is the basis to hypothesize a wider space of 'epistemic possibilities', built according to the relationship between knowledge activities and network integration. Knowledge activities can be ranked according to diversity, in a spectrum between 'focused' (with a single focus in one area, such as experiential knowledge or biomedical research) and 'diverse' or 'hybrid' (with diverse domains of engagement). Network integration can be ranked within a continuum between the two opposite poles of 'weak' and 'robust': strong and heterogenous links with other actors mean for networks to be robust. The framework contemplates four different types of organizations:

Type A: robust hybrid organizations, characterized by the production of multi-focused knowledge and robust network integration (like the patient organization cited above in its third stage of life);

Type B: weak hybrid organizations, aiming to diversify their epistemic areas, but having still limited network capacity (the case's organization in its second stage).

Type C: weak focused organizations, which focus just on one type of knowledge (disease's experiential knowledge) and are linked with only one or few networks.

Type D: robust focused organizations, are those *able to incorporate their specific, unique knowledge form as a key contribution to a wider process of knowledge making* (p. 3356).

Communication skills are critical for both written and oral communications (Brière *et al.*, 2015), especially when international relationships take place. Writing communication skills are necessary for example for setting up reports and other documents to present to key-partners and stakeholders, as well as for writing clear and unequivocal internal and external emails. Oral communication is equally important, and it does not just mean clear expression, but also ability to listen counterparts, understand their needs and preferences and avoid conflicts. In this regards, good language knowledge facilitates communication mechanisms. The European fragility of patients' organizations is also due to poor communication and language skills. On the one hand, they lack technical and bureaucratic languages used by EU institutions and national authorities; on the other side, their knowledge of English is not diffuse along the entire organizations, where only top governance levels are able to work and communicate in English. This fact can hinder the effective penetration of information and delay bottom-up responses to consultations on EU topics. It can even happen that organizations do not have suitable representatives to attend international meetings. Public speaking skills are required for any NGO's worker, in order to communicate to an ample audience key messages and initiatives. A good speaker must be entertaining, inspiring, clear and persuasive. Inner characteristics are not enough to achieve good results, since public speaking is one of those types of skills to be practiced lifelong. In preparing a speech, a NGO's worker has to adapt language to the target audience, work on her/his body language, and properly structure the speech: introduction of the key issue, description of what causes it, possible options of intervention, proposal of a valid solution to deal with the problem (https://www.etu.org.za/toolbox/docs/organise/webspeech.html).

TECHNOLOGY RELATED SKILLS

This part of the 'antenna skill framework' mainly focused two areas of skills: one related to Information and Communication Technology and the other to social media networking. The ICT skills are a basic requirement to enter in the job market (Garrido & Sullivan, 2012), required transversally by any sector (not just the information technology's) and jobs' types. The digital evolution and the social media explosion provided new opportunities for non-governmental organizations to cultivate relationships all over the globe, transcending physical boundaries and minimizing costs. The use of new media in NGOs is particularly routed to promotional scopes for NGOs' images and to aid fundraising (Seo *et al.*, 2009). Patients and professionals use social media for different motives: the first ones to find information and social support from their peers, the second ones to communicate with colleagues and for marketing reasons (Antheunis *et al.*, 2013). Through social media networking, patients' organizations can provide support to both the above categories, intermediating and 'translating' information originally provided with different scopes and languages. Social media management skills are also required to continuously engage with stakeholders, showing activities being carried out, ongoing and/or future projects, and calls for partnerships at national and international levels.

FUTURE RESEARCH DIRECTIONS

The chapter reviewed key requirements for effective management of patients' organizations, in order to let them disclose their full potential in terms of contribution to policy making, healthcare delivery, education and R&D. In pace with literature and practice on patients' organizations and general NGOs, it was proposed the 'antenna skill framework', an illustration summarizing the necessary knowledge and skills for patient organizations' management. Particular attention was devoted to management and administration skills, also proposing a business model canvas tailored to patients' organizations. Further researches should validate such frameworks through a process of stakeholders' engagement. In particular, to get comments and suggestions, and to make appropriate adjustments, it is planned the submission of the two frameworks (the 'antenna skill framework' and the tailored 'business model canvas') to patient organizations' leaders and workers, healthcare providers, policy makers, and representatives of the pharmaceutical industry. The use of inputs from these actors may lead to include more knowledge and skill areas to be developed within patients' organizations, and to re-arrange the business model canvas according to issues and challenges reported by practitioners.

Future researches should also deepen, through further literature review and relevant case studies, the potential trade-offs linked to the professionalization of patients' organizations. For example, the European Medicines Agency states that NGOs (as patients' organizations) need a certain level of professionalization to be able to work with international governmental bodies; on the contrary, it warns that greater professionalization, determining a change in one entity's internal organization and a wider engagement on not membership-focused activities, can undermine representativeness and ability to give voice to the generality of their members (Gadd, 2012). These pitfalls could be addressed in pair with other criticalities depicted by policy reports, such as lack of earmarked funding, understaffing, underdeveloped knowledge base (Sienkiewicz & Van Lingen, 2017, p. 20).

CONCLUSION

The present study has faced core knowledge and skills required for the management of patients' organizations. As NGOs representing patients' interests and aiming to improve healthcare quality and accessibility, these organizations need to present a high propensity to internal and external capacity building. Routing the analysis to the Lewis's work (2003), they are ideally learning organizations able to respond to environmental changes through a mixed managerial approach taking inspirations from business management, third sector and public management, and *an improvisational process of innovation and adaptation*. The chapter proposes the 'antenna skill framework' as an illustrative model summarizing the necessary knowledge and skills for patient organizations' management, whose building blocks are knowledge and skills' areas: about the institutional framework and its sub-systems, disease-related, technical and managerial. Each educational and training area is analyzed in relation to patient organizations' literature, and, where not available, to applicable literature about NGOs. In response to critical areas highlighted by public reports on patients' organizations, management and administration skills are targeted and deepened, also proposing an innovative business model canvas tailored to patients' organizations, blending two different versions of business model canvas focused on the not-for-profit sector and remarking multiple roles of stakeholders, potential conflicts of interests, as well as social and environmental revenues and costs. After proper validation through multi-stakeholder engagement, the frameworks presented in this chapter could represent an insightful agenda to foster policy makers, universities and other educational operators, both public and private, in conceiving suitable training programs to form capable patient managers.

REFERENCES

ALTEMS. (2018). *PAL: risultati preliminari della survey "I manager delle Associazioni pazienti tra passato, presente e futuro"*. Università Cattolica del Sacro Cuore. Retrieved August 1, 2019, from: http://www.panoramasanita.it/wp-content/uploads/2018/07/Sintesi_Survey_altems.pdf

Antheunis, M. L., Tates, K., & Nieboer, T. E. (2013). Patients' and health professionals' use of social media in healthcare: Motives, barriers and expectations. *Patient Education and Counseling*, *92*(3), 426–431. doi:10.1016/j.pec.2013.06.020 PMID:23899831

Armstrong, A., & Foley, P. (2003). Foundations of a learning organization: Organization learning mechanism. *The Learning Organization*, *10*(2), 74–82. doi:10.1108/09696470910462085

Batti, R. C. (2014). Human Resource Management Challenges Facing Local NGOs. *Humanities and Social Sciences*, *2*(4), 87–95. doi:10.11648/j.hss.20140204.11

Billis, D. (1993). *Organising Public and Voluntary Agencies*. London, UK: Routledge.

Boe, A. (1994). *Networking success: How to turn business and financial relationships into fun and profit*. Sacramento, CA: Health Communications.

Bovaird, T. (2007). Beyond Engagement and Participation: User and Community Coproduction of Public Services. *Public Administration Review*, *67*(5), 846–860. doi:10.1111/j.1540-6210.2007.00773.x

Brett, J., Staniszewska, S., Mockford, C., Herron-Marx, S., Hughes, J., Tysall, C., & Suleman, R. (2014). Mapping the impact of patient and public involvement on health and social care research: A systematic review. *Health Expectations*, *17*(5), 637–650. doi:10.1111/j.1369-7625.2012.00795.x PMID:22809132

Brière, S., Proulx, D., Navaro Flores, O., & Laporte, M. (2015). Competencies of project managers in international NGOs: Perceptions of practitioners. *International Journal of Project Management*, *33*(1), 116–125. doi:10.1016/j.ijproman.2014.04.010

Cooper, H., McMurray, A., Ward, L., & Connor, M. (2016). Implementing patient-centred care in the context of an integrated care program. *International Journal of Care Coordination*, *18*(4), 72–77. doi:10.1177/2053434516639336

De Klerk, S. (2010). The importance of networking as a management skill. *South African Journal of Business Management*, *41*(1), 37–49. doi:10.4102ajbm.v41i1.512

De Man, A. (2004). *The Networked Economy: Strategy, structure and management*. Cheltenham, UK: Edgar Elgar.

Del Fiore, L. (2016). Antonella, Patrizia e la competenza da costruire insieme. Storie di partecipazione e coinvolgimento. *Forward – Pazienti*, *3*, 2-3.

Driessen, P. P. J., Glasbergen, P., & Verdaas, C. (2001). Interactive policy-making - a model of management for public works. *European Journal of Operational Research*, *128*(2), 322–337. doi:10.1016/S0377-2217(00)00075-8

European Federation for Pharmaceutical Industries and Associations. (2011). EFPIA Code of practice on relationships between the pharmaceutical industry and patient organizations. Brussels: European Federation for Pharmaceutical Industries and Associations.

European Patients Forum. (2016). *Roadmap for Action on Patient Empowerment, European Patients Forum Work Program*. Brussels: European Patients Forum.

Fowler, A. (1997). *Striking a Balance: A Guide to Enhancing the Effectiveness of NGOs in International Development*. London, UK: Earthscan.

Gadd, C. (2012). *Professionalization and representativeness among civil society representatives*. Amsterdam: European Medicines Agency.

Garrido, M., & Sullivan, J. (2012). Understanding the Links Between ICT Skills Training and Employability: An Analytical Framework. *Information Technologies and International Development*, *8*(2), 17–32.

Hajjaj, O., & Mandysova, I. (2017). *Soft Skills Importance in NGOs' Positions.* Paper presented at the 2017 Management International Conference (MIC), Venice, Italy.

Hunter, A., Facey, K., Thomas, V., Haerry, D., Warner, K., Klingmann, I., ... See, W. (2018). EUPATI Guidance for Patient Involvement in Medicines Research and Development: Health Technology Assessment. *Frontiers in Medicine*, *5*(231), 1–10. PMID:30238004

Kara, A., Spillan, J. E., & De Shields, O. W. Jr. (2004). An Empirical Investigation of the Link Between Market Orientation and Business Performance in Non-profit Service Providers. *Journal of Marketing Theory and Practice*, *12*(2), 59–72. doi:10.1080/10696679.2004.11658519

Kay, F. (2004). *Brilliant business connections: How powerful networking can transform you and your company's performance*. Oxford, UK: How to Books.

Korten, D. C. (1987). Third Generation NGO Strategies: A Key to People-Centred Development. *World Development*, *15*(Supplement), 145–159. doi:10.1016/0305-750X(87)90153-7

Kotler, P. (1979). Strategies for Introducing Marketing into Non-profit Organizations. *Journal of Marketing*, *43*(1), 37–44. doi:10.1177/002224297904300104

Kotler, P. (1982). *Marketing for Non-profit Organizations*. Prentice Hall.

Lambell, R., Ramia, G., Nyland, C., & Michelotti, M. (2008). NGOs and international business research: Progress, prospects and problems. *International Journal of Management Reviews*, *10*(1), 75–92. doi:10.1111/j.1468-2370.2007.00218.x

Lewis, D. (2001). *The Management of Non-Governmental Development Organisations: An Introduction*. London, UK: Routledge.

Lewis, D. (2003). Theorizing the organization and management of non-governmental development organizations. *Public Management Review*, *5*(3), 325–344. doi:10.1080/1471903032000146937

Marquardt, M. J. (2011). *Building the Learning Organization: Achieving Strategic Advantage through a Commitment to Learning*. Boston, MA: Nicholas Brealey Publishing.

Moreira, T. (2014). Understanding the role of patient organizations in health technology assessment. *Health Expectations*, *18*(6), 3349–3357. doi:10.1111/hex.12325 PMID:25494707

Munns, A. K., & Bjeirmi, B. F. (1996). The role of project management in achieving project success. *International Journal of Project Management, 4*(2), 84–87.

Osterwalder, A., & Pigneur, Y. (2010). *Business model generation*. Hoboken, NJ: John Wiley & Sons.

Padanyi, P., & Gainer, B. (2004). Market Orientation in the Nonprofit Sector: Taking Multiple Constituencies into Consideration. *Journal of Marketing Theory and Practice, 12*(2), 43–58. doi:10.1080/10696679.2004.11658518

Power, J., & Waddell, D. (2004). The link between self-managed work teams and learning organizations using performance indicators. *The Learning Organization, 11*(3), 244–259. doi:10.1108/09696470410533003

Rathert, C., Huddleston, N., & Pak, Y. (2011). Acute care patients discuss the patient role in patient safety. *Health Care Management Review, 36*(2), 134–144. doi:10.1097/HMR.0b013e318208cd31 PMID:21317659

Rathert, C., Wyrwich, M. D., & Boren, S. A. (2013). Patient-centered care and outcomes a systematic review of the literature. *Medical Care Research and Review: MCRR, 70*(4), 351–379. doi:10.1177/1077558712465774 PMID:23169897

Rebelo, T. M., & Gomes, A. D. (2011). Conditioning factors of an organizational learning culture. *Journal of Workplace Learning, 23*(3), 173–194. doi:10.1108/13665621111117215

Robinson, T., Clemson, B., & Keating, C. (1997). Development of high organizational learning units. *The Learning Organization, 4*(5), 228–234. doi:10.1108/09696479710186412

Salamon, L., & Anheier, H. (1999). The Third Sector in the Third World. In D. Lewis (Ed.), *International Perspectives on Voluntary Action: Reshaping the Third Sector*. London, UK: Earthscan.

Salamon, L. M., & Anheier, H. K. (1996). *The international classification of nonprofit organizations ICNPO Revision 1, Working Papers of the Johns Hopkins Comparative Nonprofit Sector Project, n. 19*. Baltimore, MD: The Johns Hopkins Institute for Policy Studies.

Sargeant, A., Foreman, S., & Liao, M. (2002). Operationalizing the Marketing Concept in the Nonprofit Sector. *Journal of Nonprofit & Public Sector Marketing, 10*(2), 41–65. doi:10.1300/J054v10n02_03

Selby, J. V., & Lipstein, S. H. (2014). PCORI at 3 years. Progress, lessons, and plans. *The New England Journal of Medicine, 370*(7), 592–595. doi:10.1056/NEJMp1313061 PMID:24521104

Senge, P. M. (1990). *The fifth discipline: The art and practice of learning organization*. New York, NY: Doubleday.

Seo, H., Kim, J. Y., & Yang, S. (2009). Global activism and new media: A study of transnational NGOs' online public relations. *Public Relations Review, 35*(2), 123–126. doi:10.1016/j.pubrev.2009.02.002

Sienkiewicz, D., & Van Lingen, C. (2017). *The Added Value of Patient Organisations, Report EPF European Patients Forum Work Program*. Brussels: European Patients Forum.

Stanley, V. G., & Albin, G. J. (2013). Challenges for human resource experts in global scenarios. *International Journal of Advancements in Research & Technology, 2*(4), 209–214.

Tsang, E. W. K. (1997). Organizational Learning and the Learning Organization: A Dichotomy between Descriptive and Prescriptive Research. *Human Relations, 50*(1), 73–89. doi:10.1177/001872679705000104

Watkins, K. E., & Marsick, V. J. (1999). *Facilitating Learning Organizations: Making Learning Count.* Gower Publishing Limited.

Weinberger, D. (2011). *Too Big to Know: Rethinking Knowledge Now That the Facts Aren't the Facts, Experts Are Everywhere, and the Smartest Person in the Room*. New York, NY: Basic Books.

KEY TERMS AND DEFINITIONS

Business Model Canvas: Framework to represent how strategies can be implemented within an organization. The original version was developed for for-profit businesses and it is made of nine building blocks (customer segments, value propositions, channels, customer relationships, revenue streams, key resources, key activities, key partnerships, cost structure). In a not-for-profit version, the business model canvas contains two more building blocks (social and environmental costs, and social and environmental revenues).

Fundraising: Activity of requiring financial support to public and private actors. It normally constitutes the principal source of revenues for non-profit organizations, driven by a fundraising plan establishing the desired amount of money to collect, the funding sources, the related fundraising initiatives (and timelines) that the organization will undertake, as well as an estimation of the costs associated to them.

Learning Organizations: Organizations where people collectively learn how to learn, continually developing new patterns of thinking and the capacity to achieve desired results. They are characterized by seven interrelated dimensions: continuous learning, dialogue and inquiry, team learning, embedded system, system connections, empowerment and leadership. The ability of such organizations to adapt to environmental changes makes them innovative and performing.

NGOs: Acronym for non-governmental organizations. Entities being part of the third sector, not belonging neither to government constituencies nor to the for-profit sector. Their distinctive features are: organization (institutionalized and retaining a persistent internal organizational structure), private origin (have an institutional identity separate from that of the government's apparatus), self-governance (equipped to control their own activities through internal governance procedures); non-profit orientation (they do not distribute profits and reinvest them into activities related to the mission of the organization), voluntarism (engage volunteers in management and operations, with non-compulsory memberships).

Planning and Control: Management function consisting on (1) setting in advance organizational objectives (strategic, tactic, operational), (2) planning how to achieve them, and (3) monitoring the level of fulfillment of objectives (both during implementation and afterwards), in order to analyze the causal tissue of gaps and undertake corrective actions. Planning and control activities require synergies between accounting systems and performance measurement systems.

Skill: The ability to apply knowledge and use know-how to complete tasks and solve problems.

Chapter 5
The Potential of System Dynamics to Model Patient-Aided Healthcare

ABSTRACT

This chapter explores the potential of system dynamics (or SD), a computer-aided methodology for policy analysis and design, to investigate patient organizations' contribution to healthcare. The chapter starts by describing the complexity features of the healthcare sector. Then it illustrates SD building blocks. A literature review of previous system dynamics applications to healthcare care issues categorizes selected papers according to relevant criteria. It emerges that few models incorporate patients' characteristics and perspective, none of them specifically dealing with patients' organizations and patient co-created health. In conclusion, the chapter highlights how SD can be considered a suitable methodology to depict the outcome of patients and their organizations' participation to healthcare processes, filling a gap in literature about both qualitative and quantitative system dynamics.

BACKGROUND

Patients' organizations are actors belonging to the third sector and operating within healthcare. The latter is a system characterized by complexity, because of the relevant number of interrelated actors, variables and processes, involving many aspects, included organizational leadership, management and decision-

DOI: 10.4018/978-1-7998-2653-8.ch005

making (Plsek & Greenhalgh, 2001). Thus, it is opinion of the chapter' author that studying these organizations cannot neglect the complexity of the health system (Bar-Yam, 2006; Patel & Cohen, 2008; Plsek & Greenhalgh, 2001) in which they are embedded.

Such complexity is exacerbated by new technologies and the increasing consumer expectations and awareness of health issues, which put pressure on practitioners of all disciplines and healthcare organizations to *accommodate innovation and simultaneously ensure that their current practices are effective, safe and efficient* (Forbes, & Griffith, 2002, p. 141). Notwithstanding, there can be registered failures to adopt innovations even when supported by sound evidence, or, at the contrary, the perseverance of ineffective practices (Sackett *et al.*, 1998). In fact, evidence-based healthcare, although useful to ensure that medical practice is aligned with current best evidence, is affected by limitations, since it just focuses on evidence from randomized controlled trials, neglecting information generated by qualitative research or by the experience of practitioners themselves (Pawson, 2002). According to scholars, evidence-based medicine is not in contradiction with patient-centered practices (Epstein & Street, 2011) and with shared decision making (Hoffman *et al.*, 2014). In this stream, evidence-based medicine and shared decision making are two essential and complementary aspects for the delivery of quality healthcare, albeit the processes of patient integration in the clinical choices are still poorly mapped and scarce attention is devoted to them (Hoffman *et al.*, 2014). However, despite the today's sensibility to these themes, patients still result substantially excluded by the decisions regarding their health (Barry & Edgman-Levitan, 2012).

On the other side, medicine is traditionally founded on classical reductionism, where a certain problem is broken down into its smallest components, examined, and then the retained information used to draw conclusions about the nature of the larger reality (Tuffin, 2016). Such an approach is successful for linear systems, i.e. systems characterized by relatively low complexity and predictable and proportional behaviors in response to external influences (Plsek & Greenhalgh, 2001). Conversely, the complexity paradigm, based on systems theory, informatics and cybernetics, investigates the healthcare as a complex adaptive system (Fajardo-Ortiz *et al.*, 2015). Far from the reductionist healthcare epistemology, it presents a broad conceptualization to understand complex systems (no matter if they are physical, biological or social), sharing the same characteristics. According to Kannampallil and colleagues (2011) interrelatedness, meaning that system components influence each other, is a key property defining complex systems and the level of their complexity.

Then the complexity of a healthcare system increases with the number of its components, the relations between them, and the uniqueness of those relations. This latter signifies that expanding a system by mere repetition of relations and components does not substantively increase its complexity. From interrelatedness descend other complexity properties, such as non-decomposability, emergence and nonlinear behaviors. Non-decomposability means that a complex system, like the healthcare one, cannot be understood by looking at isolated components, but at substantially interrelated ones. Emergence means that interactions between components of complex systems often lead to systems' unexpected behavioral properties, resulting from the system's self-organization processes and complicating system responses to external influences (Fajardo-Ortiz *et al.*, 2015).

Differently from relatively simple systems, characterized by linearities, complex systems tend to nonlinear behaviors, i.e. they do not behave predictably and proportionately (Plsek & Greenhalgh, 2001). Moreover, complex systems constantly change and hold high sensitivity to initial conditions, so that systems with similar or same structures can witness very different behavior patterns due to differences (sometimes slight) in initial parameters. They are related with time because of trade-offs between long- and short-term effects of decisions, which must be taken into consideration during service planning and control (Fajardo-Ortiz et al. 2015). Finally, most complex systems are characterized by relative mathematical simplicity, i.e. they are governed and can be explained by relatively simple mathematical equations or 'rules' (Tuffin, 2016).

Given the above discourse, the study of healthcare issues requires cognitive and computational efforts rejecting any reductionism and rather requiring systemic, inter-institutional and interdisciplinary approaches. Among the investigation approaches grounded in system theory and cybernetics, this chapter explores the potential of system dynamics in dealing with patient organizations' contribution to healthcare. System dynamics (or SD) is a simulation methodology able to aid policy design and analysis. Originally developed by Jay Forrester (1961) to face industrial dynamics, over the time has been applied to many fields (e.g. Coyle, 2000; Xing & Dangerfield, 2018). The decision to route healthcare research to system dynamics is because SD fits the case of complex systems with interdependences, mutual interactions, information feedbacks, temporal delays, and circular causality (Richardson, 1991). Thus, the possible issues that can be proficiently handed by SD can belong to socio-economic, managerial or biological systems. In the next paragraphs, there will be illustrated the system dynamics building blocks and a literature review of previous applications to healthcare.

ADOPTING SYSTEM DYNAMICS TO FACE THE COMPLEXITY OF HEALTHCARE

System Dynamics Modelling

System dynamics is a methodology aided by computer modelling and simulations, suitable to deal with dynamic problems (issue behaviors occurring over the time) in complex social, economic or ecological systems, characterized by interdependences, mutual interactions, information feedbacks, temporal delays, and circular causality (Richardson, 1991). SD models are built according to a certain guiding philosophy and require the design of two kinds of diagrams: stock-and-flow and causal loops. A stock-and-flow structure is a map of a certain problem's causal tissue, tracking processes of accumulation of material, information and money in a network of stocks, flows and information feedbacks (Sterman, 2000).

Stocks are the level of accumulation of resources, measured by punctual quantities or amounts in a certain moment, conventionally denoted by rectangles. Flows are the rates making stocks to change over time, measured by quantities or amounts occurring in the time unit and denoted by pipes inflowing or outflowing the stocks. In addition to stocks and flows, a model includes auxiliary variables, denoted by circles. The latter can have a twofold function: they can help calculus through ratios and other mathematical constructs, or they can bring constant or exogenous parameters to the model.

The stock-and-flow structure has a mathematic root, since it discloses a set of differential equations, with derivatives taking place in pace with time. Indeed, time is discretized into intervals of length dt, and SD software packages simulate behavior patterns one interval at a time. As a result, the level of a stock at time t, is the result of its value at time (t - dt) and its net rate of change, difference between the inflows and the outflows respectively feeding and draining the stock in the chosen time step (Richardson 1991). Each stock, besides constants and exogenous parameters, can impact on the flows connected to the other stocks, directly or through auxiliary variables. The general equation for a stock variable is as follows.

$$\text{STOCK(t)} = \text{STOCK(t-dt)} + \text{dt} * \text{NET RATE OF CHANGE (t-dt)} \quad (1)$$

There no exist a general equation for flows, which can be formalized with maths involving other flows, stocks, converters, or estimated parameters or constants. Sometimes modelers prefer to not to separate inflows and outflows, and use a synthetic flow structures, the bi-flows, directly expressive of stocks' net rates of change (Sterman, 2000).

A simple stock-and-flow diagram is portrayed in figure 1. The stock 1 results from the accumulation of differences between its inflow and outflow over time. The inflow depends on three auxiliary variables, denoted with numbers 1, 2 and 5. The outflow is affected by stock 1 and auxiliary 4. It is possible to notice that variable 1 and 4 are exogenous, i.e. they are kept at the boundaries of the model and are not affected by any other influence within the model structure. All the other auxiliaries take part to the relevant system's causal tissue, affecting and being affected by other variables. For example, auxiliary 2, influenced by stock 1, impacts on auxiliary 3, in turn modifying the bi-flow to stock 2. The latter influences variable 5, which feeds back to the first stock's inflow.

Another SD tool to represent the feedback structure of a model is the causal loop diagram. It consists of a network of loops mutually interacting within the relevant system and reflecting the endogeneity of the system dynamics models (Richardson, 2011), where the structure causes problematic behaviors to arise. A simplified causal loop diagram is sketched in figure 2 and shows the interplay of two different loops. The variables are linked by arrows connoted by polarities. The 'plus' means that there is a positive link: if a certain variable increases, the linked variable *ceteris paribus* increases as well; on the contrary, if the first variable diminishes, the second variable diminishes too. The 'minus' represents a negative relation: a raise in a variable this time determines a reduction in the other variable. Following figure 2, there is a positive link between variables X and Y, Y and X, X and Y, whilst the link between Y and Z is negative, i.e. with changes occurring, *ceteris paribus*, in opposite directions.

The models' dynamics are the result of the interactions of feedback loops, which can assume two possible connotations:

1. Reinforcing or positive loops: they tend to enhance initial conditions, provoking virtuous or vicious mechanisms of growth or decay (loop R in figure 2).

Figure 1. Example of a stock-and-flow diagram

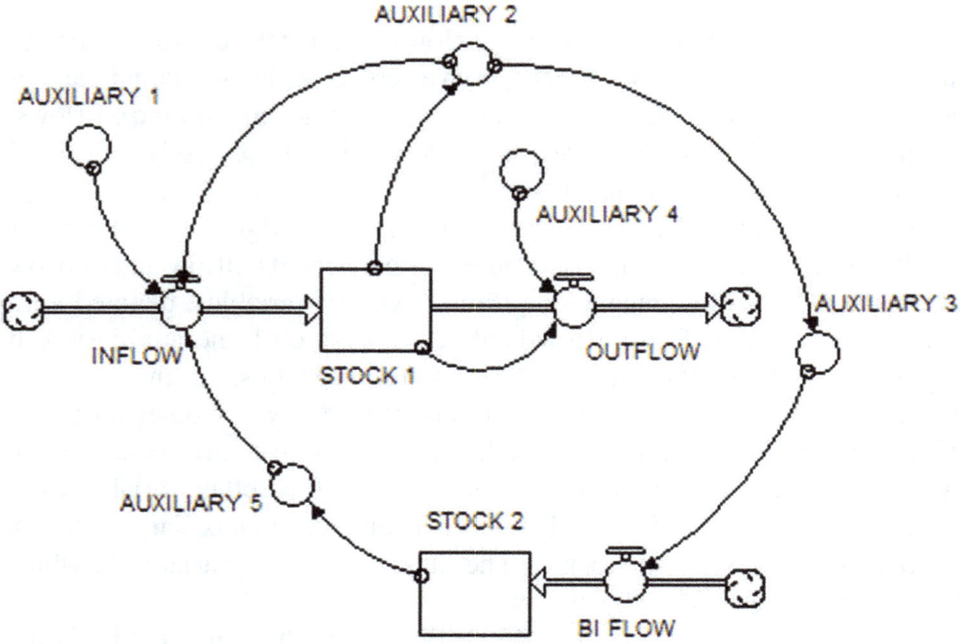

Figure 2. Example of causal loop diagram

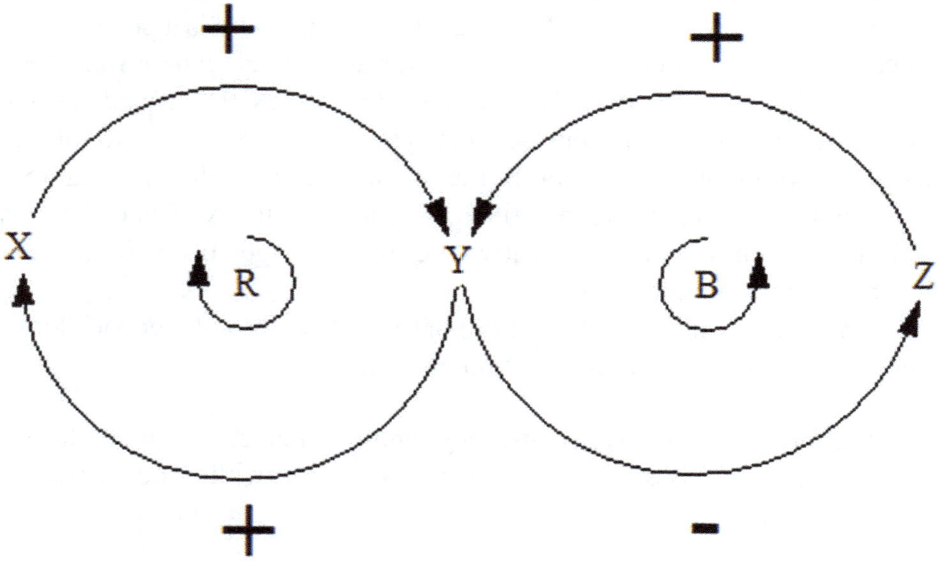

2. Balancing or negative loops: they tend to equilibrate the system dynamics, or to stabilize the initial conditions, or to let the system approach a certain goal (loop B in figure 2).

The loop polarity is determined by the multiplication of the signs of every single link belonging to the loop or, that is the same, accounting the number of negative links within the loop, which is odd for balancing loops and even for reinforcing loops. Thus, the adjectives positive and negative, (referable both to links and loops), do not state for goodness of the related dynamics, but they are just conventional features of SD models.

Stock-and-flow and causal loop structures represent outputs of system dynamics qualitative modelling. However, SD potential is fully developed whenever the modelling efforts lead to quantitative formalization, model calibration and performing of simulations. A simulation software (for example, Ithink by Stella) provides users with the possibility to progressively build the stock-and-flow structure and contemporary insert equations representative of decision rules and behavioral relationships. Then, the quantitative model is tested to check if the relevant variables' simulated patterns fit the historical ones within the same causal tissue. At that point, it is possible to use simulations to test the behavior of the system according to the activation of policy levers.

SD software's interface also gives the opportunity to build control panels, like the one in figure 3, where the activation of alternative policies relates to time series of problematic behaviors. In the example, it is graphed a generic 'problematic behavior pattern', portrayed in line 1. This could be, for example, rising costs to provide a certain service, not paired with adequate level of quality. Three policy measures have been conceived and their potential impacts are simulated along a 24-quarters timeframe. Policy 3 appears the best suited in comparison with the other options, and this simulation may induce decision-makers to further explore the feasibility of this choice.

Modelling Paths

Using the SD tools, it is possible to imagine 4 basic modelling paths, characterized by growing complexity, whose main steps are illustrated in figure 4. On the left side, there are qualitative modelling paths; on the right, modelling paths mixing qualitative and quantitative SD modelling.

In path 1, the causal loop diagram is the first modelling output, followed by stock-and-flow structures progressively enriching the feedback analysis with the definition of accumulation processes. This is a qualitative modelling,

Figure 3. Example of control panel for system dynamics simulations

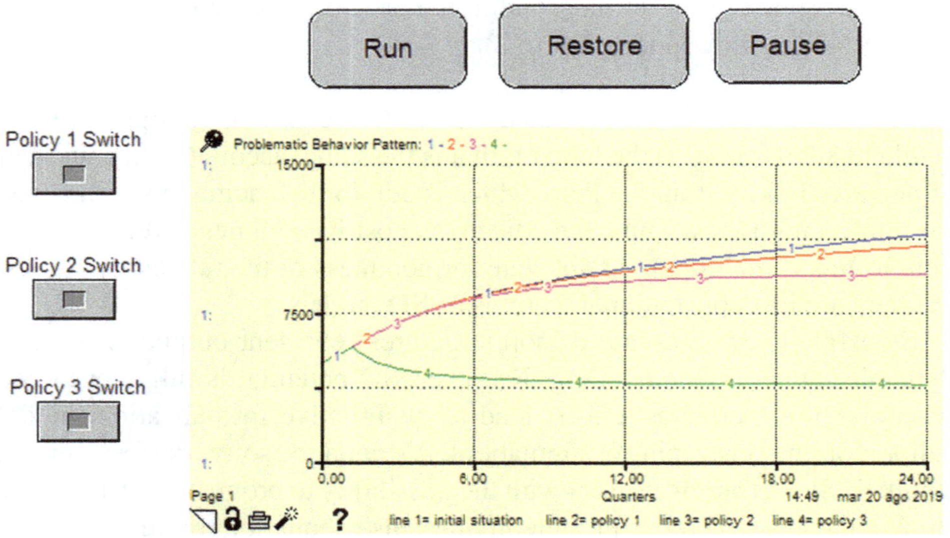

used to map dynamic causal hypotheses according to different sources of literature, or causal influences in stakeholders' or modelers' views, or both things. This way to proceed could be used for qualitative researches or as an intermediate phase of quantitative researches (path 3), or it can happen that a research initially conceived as purely qualitative is switched to quantitative, so that path 1 is enlarged towards quantitative connotations.

In path 2, the qualitative modelling starts by portraying the stock-and-flow structure, based on which key causal loops are identified to provide hypothetical explanations to dynamic problems. This path, albeit qualitative like the previous one, has a more synthetic approach: from a wider structure of accumulation processes it selects key variables responsible for the system's feedback structure. Even in this case, the path can be used for qualitative researches or as an intermediate phase of quantitative researches (path 4).

In the third modelling path, preliminary causal loops allow to sketch key variables and mutual influences. These maps are progressively enriched and specified with stock-and-flow structures. Then the quantitative modelling starts through the construction of equations, iterative simulations, parameter and sensitivity testing and new inputs from literature and from empirical researches. By mean of iterative trials and errors in simulations, the modeler's understanding of the problem proceeds, thus new adjustments are made, first on the stock-and-flow structures and then to the causal loops.

Figure 4. Alternative modelling paths

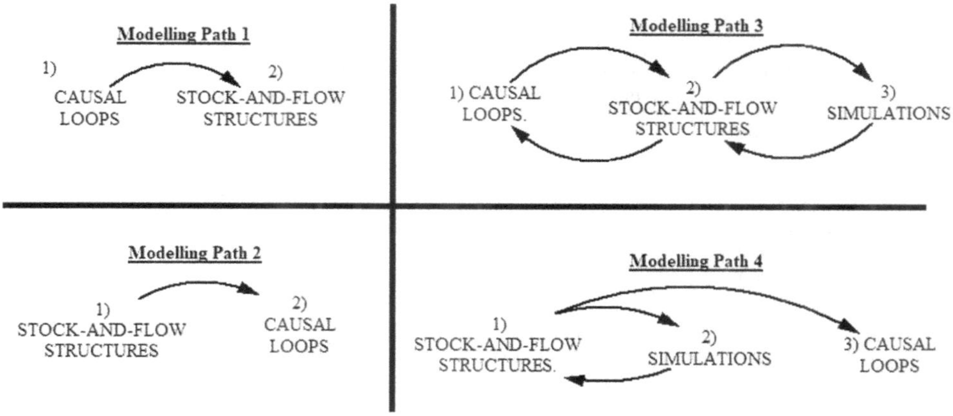

The last path starts by the progressive building of stock-and-flow diagrams, aided by computer simulations able to suggest changes to the model structure. Once the quantitative model is complete, causal loop diagrams are sketched to perform further model analyses.

LITERATURE REVIEW ON HEALTHCARE APPLICATIONS

This section of the chapter is devoted to a description of system dynamics applications to healthcare issues. The selection was done by doing Boolean researches of the words 'system dynamics + health', first scanning of abstracts, selection of papers whose texts going through, final inclusion of papers. This process led to the selection of 33 papers, categorized in table 1.

In the horizontal axis, some model features are highlighted. Model contained into the papers are firstly distinguished according to their use of macro or micro modelling. The latter depends on the amplitude of model boundaries, referred respectively to the healthcare system as a whole and to an organizational level. Then papers explicitly modelling patients' characteristics (epidemiological, behavioral) and investigating patients' perspective are counted.

In the vertical axis, papers are distinguished according to the SD stage in which their dynamic models lay. It is accounted if the paper makes use just of causal loop diagrams (CLD), stock-and-flows (SFD) and simulations. It is worth noticing that in one case the paper contained two different models considered relevant for this study, that's why the total amount of models (spread

Table 1. Synthesis of literature on SD applications according to selected criteria

MODEL FEATURES/ MODELLING STAGE	MACRO-MODELLING (Healthcare systems' level)	MICRO-MODELLING (Organizational level)	Explicitly modelled patients' characteristics	Investigated patients' perspective
Causal Loop Diagramming (CLD)	7	-	2	1
Stock-and-flow Diagramming (SFD)	4	-	1	-
Simulations (eventually paired with CLD and/or SFD)	19	4	5	-
TOT	30	4	8	1

in micro and macro modelling along the modelling stages) is 34, instead of 33. In general, papers bringing quantitative modelling outputs (simulations) also contained at least a qualitative diagram (CLD or SFD).

The system dynamics literature highlights the massive presence of macro models (30 models over 34), i.e. models portraying healthcare issues at level of national or local healthcare systems. Most of them (23 models) are quantitative and present simulated scenario analyses. As far as macro-models are concerned, the application types are several. A first kind of models targets hospital systems. For example, Wolstenholme (1999) applies SD to the development of UK policy guidelines. He proposes a model of total patient flows to test alternative policy measures, among which the implementation of intermediate care facilities can reduce waiting lists more than canonical solutions such as an increase of bed capacity. The same author, in collaboration with other colleagues (Wolstenholme *et al.,* 2007), proposes for the same context the 'delayed hospital discharge model', a comprehensive structure made of the following sectors: hospitals, care at home, intermediate care, rehab and interim care.

Hirsch *et al.* (2012) propose simulation modelling focusing US local health systems. Other models target healthcare systems congested by high emergency admission rates. A first model (Brailsford *et al.*, 2004) simulates patient flows and system bottlenecks within the UK context, showing the positive effect of preventing emergency admissions for elderly population, reducing bed occupancy. A paper of Royston *et al.* (1999) proposes two SD applications. The first one evaluates the potential impact of screening policies for cervical cancer and chlamydia. The second model proposes qualitative SFD with the aim to develop emergency care. Abo-Hamas and his colleagues (2015) built a quantitative model to address the Irish healthcare system congestion, ascribable to the overcrowding of emergency departments. Lattimer *et al.* (2004) built an SD model on emergency and urgent care. The model, populated with demographic and activity data, simulates patterns of demand and system bottlenecks in pace with alternative policy options to mitigate the problem.

Wolstenholme (1993) also emphasizes the usefulness of system dynamics qualitative models, by mean of a case study in community care. Diaz and others (2012) use SD quantitative modelling for resource planning and utilization within US ambulatory healthcare service. Other modeling efforts have been made to address specific pathologies: e.g. chronic diseases (Homer et al. 2004; 2006; Loyo et al., 2012), depressive disorders (Wittenborn *et al.*, 2015), obesity (Fallah-Fini & Rahmandad, 2014). Marshall *et al.* (2010) built a stock-and-flow structure to deal with osteoarthritis in the Canadian context. Rwashana *et al.* (2009) proposes a simulation model about a Ugandan case study, portraying the dynamic influences associated with demand and provision of immunization services. Chalmers and colleagues (2009) use quantitative SD to justify pharmacotherapy policy decisions adopted by the Australian National Council on Drugs. Cavana & Tobias (2009) use system dynamics to assist the New Zealand Ministry of Health in the evaluation of tobacco control policies, such as the introduction of less addictive or less toxic cigarettes.

A big stream of healthcare applications refers to pure managerial issues. Merrill *et al.* (2013) build causal loop diagrams to evaluate the implementation dynamics of an electronic health information reporting system at the New York State Department of Health. Mehrjerdi (2012) proposes a quantitative SD model to show interconnections between weight factor, health problems and expenses to be paid by insurance companies (spread into operational expenses and expenses for treatment, medication, hospitality and drug treatment). Masnick & McDonnell (2010), in order to help healthcare service planners in decision making about service workforce and skill mix, build a stock-and-flow structure putting together clinical workforce, workloads, technologies, productivity and quality issues. Barber & Lopez-Valcarel (2010), facing the problem of medical doctors' shortage in Spain, construct a model that combines population growth and deficits of medical specialties, suggesting an increase in the number of students admitted to medical schools.

Less diffuse were system dynamics applications targeting specific hospitals or departments, what was called micro-modelling in the present chapter. Samuel and his colleagues (2010), considering healthcare as a typical service-oriented supply chain, adopt a dynamic simulation model to examine health service supply chain systems, and proposes as policy options to reduce process stages and to make capacity adjustments. Lane (*et al.*, 2000), targeting long waiting times for admissions within accident and emergency units, models the interaction between demand, resource deployment, other hospital processes and beds. The model shows that a beds' decrease does not increase emergency admissions' delays but makes elective admissions to reduce; and while remarking the unavoidability of certain delays, argues that improvements can be obtained by increasing selected resources impacting on the accident and emergency unit. Abuhay and colleagues (2016) present a SD model to simulate congestion within a specialized medical center, due to emergency patient flows with acute coronary syndrome. Maliapen & Dangerfield (2010) develop system dynamics-based clinical pathways in an Australian hospital, with the aim to help in caseloads' redistribution.

The system dynamics literature reviewed about applications to healthcare also revealed that 8 model explicitly formalized patient characteristics, building articulated model structures other than the simple consideration of patients as exogenous demand inputs for healthcare services. Even in this regard, the quantitative modelling prevails with 5 applications, followed by one stock-and-flow diagram and 2 causal loops. So far, just one qualitative model, authored by Faezipour & Ferreira (2013) investigates patient perspective in healthcare. Starting by the need of sustainability of healthcare systems, put under pressure by diminishing resources and increasing demand, the application points out patient satisfaction as a key element of healthcare systems' social aspect. For this reason, the modelers propose a causal loop diagram, the 'patient satisfaction sustainability model', linking variables such as: patients' level of satisfaction, demand for healthcare services, accessibility, effectiveness and well-being.

Outlining System Dynamics Applications to Patient-Aided Healthcare

Given the above investigation, system dynamics methodology appears to be a suitable modelling methodology to drive researches on patient-aided healthcare. The adoption of SD would foster a better understanding of problems, impacts of alternative policy options, potential trade-offs between long term and short-term policy effects, unintended consequence of myopic decision-making, as well as the social communication of these figures. However, doing other Boolean researches of the words 'system dynamics + patient + health co-creation', and 'system dynamics + patient organizations' it has emerged that no SD application exists on patient co-created healthcare and on patient organizations' contributions to healthcare processes. Then it is possible to fill this gap in SD literature, by outlining dynamic models able to capture active contributions of patients to health processes.

Such modelling efforts should address real case studies (Yin, 2003), by proposing explanatory researches mixing qualitative and quantitative dynamic modelling, to target the dynamics of a selected patients' organization. The guiding research philosophy should mix: interpretivism (Collins, 2010, p. 38) because it aims to reach a better understanding about a complex, social, time-and-context related problem; pragmatism, because it would integrate system dynamics with suitable means, considered appropriate according to the investigated circumstances (Alford & Hughes, 2008, p. 132); and interventism (Johnsson & Lukka, 2006) in order to make both theoretical and organizational contributions, by assisting organizations in implementing changes (Dumay, 2010, p. 47).

The research approach should be devoted to the explicit pursue of public value creation by mean of a multi-stakeholder involvement, like the participative process of building system dynamics models at strategic level, suggested by Stave for environmental decisions (2002) and water management (2003). In the healthcare, tentative adoptions of group SD model building have been made by Vennix *et al.* (1994), involving VT Medicaid experts and stakeholders; by Ackermann *et al.* (2010), who organized group mapping sessions to address issues of service capacity for the provision of long term dementia services in the Scottish context; and by Merril *et al.* (2012), in coping with the implementation of electronic health information exchange for public health reporting at a state health department.

The case study could privilege macro or micro modelling, depending on the modelling purposes and the investigated objects, which could be European, national or regional healthcare policy making, research and development, or specific healthcare delivery processes, performed by hospital or community care providers, or their departments/operational units. In any case, the privileged modelling paths could be the ones mixing qualitative and quantitative modelling, i.e. paths 3 and 4, portrayed in the right side of figure 4. The reason of such preference is because the quantitative formalization of models allows a greater number of iterations and continuous improvements of the dynamic model hypothesis. However, the effective decision to integrate qualitative and quantitative modelling will also depend on available time and data for research projects. The decision to start modelling activities from causal loop or stock-and-flow diagramming will depend on the modeler's preferences.

If the modeler aims to gradually and separately integrate stakeholders 'mental models' (Doyle & Ford, 1998; 1999), She/He can use data from interviews and questionnaires to build an SFD and progressively enrich it as soon as Her/His understanding of the topic will advance. Alternatively, it could be sketched a simple causal loop according to literature findings, and relevant actors could be asked to evaluate it and to suggest adjustments and additions. Other way is to organize group model building sections where different actors may make explicit their mental models and, with the help of a system dynamics facilitator, could create major feedback loop diagrams expressive of a shared understanding of social, financial and ecological issues.

FUTURE RESEARCH DIRECTIONS

This chapter deals with the potential of system dynamics to drive researches on patient-aided healthcare, identifying a literature gap regarding SD applications on patients' organizations and processes of co-created healthcare. Future researches should address this gap by proposing case studies involving policy makers, clinicians, patients and their representative organizations, to track value creation processes, bottlenecks and opportunities. New advancements could also apply to patient co-created healthcare a group model building approach, organizing working sessions where key stakeholders could interact and, by mean of a modeler facilitator, transfer their understanding of certain issues in shared and collaborative models. Other directions of investigation may target the communication of healthcare policies to the wider social community, the identification of policies' unintended consequences and their impacts on political and social consensus.

CONCLUSION

This chapter have made a wide analysis of the potential of system dynamics to address patient-aided healthcare, with specific focus on the contribution of patients' organizations. The process was undertaken by gradual approximations. First, it was analysed the contextual complexity in which patients' organizations are embedded. In this regard, it was pointed out how the complexity approach, grounded in system theory and cybernetics, and overcoming the traditional reductionist medicine, is suitable to deal with the healthcare sector, characterized by several actors, processes and variables. Among the features of complex systems, it was reported the interrelatedness of components as the key property, able to define complex systems and from which other qualifications descend.

System dynamics modelling was chosen because of its common routes (systems and cybernetics) with complex theory, and because of its applicative flexibility. Indeed, it was remarked how SD fits any dynamic problem occurring over the time in complex systems, which could be physical, social or economic and financial. The chapter introduced and described modelling tools (causal loops, stock-and-flow diagrams, simulations) and distinguished between qualitative and quantitative modelling. Possible modelling paths have been sketched according to the order in which SD tools are iteratively used.

Then a literature review on system dynamics applications to healthcare has been proposed. A selection of articles has been categorized according to the amplitude of the modelling purposes and the qualitative or quantitative modelling approaches. Most papers contain macro-models, targeting healthcare issues from the comprehensive point of view of national or local health authorities, and privilege quantitative simulation to test, in a relatively risk-free environment, the potential impact of alternative policy options. The literature review highlighted few papers containing explicit model structures regarding patients (other than considering them as exogenous or constant input variables), and just one of them investigated healthcare from a patient perspective. Furthermore, none of the models specifically deals with patients' organizations and patient co-created healthcare. In conclusion, this chapter shows that SD can be considered a suitable methodology to depict the outcomes of patient-helped healthcare, filling a gap in literature about both qualitative and quantitative applications of system dynamics.

REFERENCES

Abo-Hamas, W., Rashwan, W., & Arisha, A. (2015). A System Dynamics View of the Acute Bed Blockage Problem in the Irish Healthcare System. *European Journal of Operational Research*, *247*(1), 276–293. doi:10.1016/j.ejor.2015.05.043

Abuhay, T. M., Krikunov, A. V., Bolgova, E. V., Ratova, L. G., & Kovalchuk, S. V. (2016). Simulation of patient flow and load of departments in a specialized medical center. *Procedia Computer Science*, *101*, 143–151. doi:10.1016/j.procs.2016.11.018

Ackermann, F., Eden, C., Andersen, D. F., & Richardson, G. P. (2010). Scripts map: A Tool for Designing Multi-method Policy-making Workshops. *Omega*, *39*(October), 427–434.

Bar-Yam, Y. (2006). Improving the effectiveness of healthcare and public health: A multiscale complex systems analysis. *American Journal of Public Health*, *96*(3), 459–466. doi:10.2105/AJPH.2005.064444 PMID:16449583

Barber, P., & Lopez-Valcarel, B. G. (2010). Forecasting the need for medical specialists in Spain: Application of a system dynamics model. *Human Resources for Health*, *8*(1), 24–32. doi:10.1186/1478-4491-8-24 PMID:21034458

Barry, M. J., & Edgman-Levitan, S. P. A. (2012). Shared Decision Making—The Pinnacle of Patient-Centered Care. *The New England Journal of Medicine*, *366*(9), 780–781. doi:10.1056/NEJMp1109283 PMID:22375967

Brailsford, S. C., Lattimer, V. A., Tarnaras, P., & Turnbull, J. C. (2004). Emergency and on-demand healthcare: Modelling a large complex system. *The Journal of the Operational Research Society*, *55*(1), 34–42. doi:10.1057/palgrave.jors.2601667

Cavana, R. Y., & Tobias, M. (2009). Integrative system dynamics: Analysis of policy options for tobacco control in New Zealand. *Behavioral Science*, *25*(5), 675–694.

Chalmers, J., Ritter, A., Heffernan, N., & McDonnel, G. (2009). Modelling pharmacotherapy maintenance in Australia. Canberra, Australia: Australia National Council on Drugs.

Collins, H. (2010). *Creative Research: The Theory and Practice of Research for the Creative Industries*. London, UK: AVA Publications.

Coyle, G. (2000). Qualitative and quantitative modelling in system dynamics: Some research questions. *System Dynamics Review*, *16*(3), 225–244. doi:10.1002/1099-1727(200023)16:3<225::AID-SDR195>3.0.CO;2-D

Diaz, R., Behr, J. G., & Tulpule, M. (2012). A system dynamics model for simulating ambulatory healthcare demands. *Simulation in Healthcare*, *7*(4), 243–250. doi:10.1097/SIH.0b013e318259d134 PMID:22722706

Doyle, J., & Ford, D. (1998). Mental models concepts for system dynamics research. *System Dynamics Review*, *14*(1), 3–29. doi:10.1002/(SICI)1099-1727(199821)14:1<3::AID-SDR140>3.0.CO;2-K

Doyle, J., & Ford, D. (1999). Mental models concepts revised: Some clarifications and a reply to Lane. *System Dynamics Review*, *15*(4), 411–415. doi:10.1002/(SICI)1099-1727(199924)15:4<411::AID-SDR181>3.0.CO;2-R

Dumay, J. C. (2010). A critical reflective discourse of an interventionist research project. *Qualitative Research in Accounting & Management*, *7*(1), 46–70. doi:10.1108/11766091011034271

Epstein, R. M., & Street, R. L. (2011). The Values and Value of Patient-Centered Care. *Annals of Family Medicine*, *9*(2), 100–103. doi:10.1370/afm.1239 PMID:21403134

Fajardo-Ortiz, G., Fernández-Ortega, M. A., Ortiz-Montalvo, A., & Olivares-Santos, R. A. (2015). The dimension of the paradigm of complexity in health systems. *Cirugia y Cirujanos*, *83*(1), 81–86. doi:10.1016/j.circir.2014.03.001 PMID:25982615

Fallah-Fini, S., Rahmandad, H., Huang, T. T.-K., Bures, R. M., & Glass, T. A. (2014). Modeling US Adult Obesity Trends: A System Dynamics Model for Estimating Energy Imbalance Gap. *American Journal of Public Health*, *104*(7), 1230–1239. doi:10.2105/AJPH.2014.301882 PMID:24832405

Forbes, A., & Griffith, P. (2002). Methodological strategies for the identification and synthesis of 'evidence' to support decision-making in relation to complex healthcare systems and practices. *Nursing Inquiry*, *9*(3), 141–155. doi:10.1046/j.1440-1800.2002.00146.x PMID:12199878

Forrester, J. W. (1961). *Industrial Dynamics*. Boston, MA: The MIT Press.

Hirsch, G., Homer, J., Milstein, B., Scherrer, L., Ingersoll, C., Landy, L., …, Fisher, E. (2012). *ReThink Health Dynamics: Understanding and Influencing Local Health System Change*. Paper presented at the 30th International Conference of the System Dynamics Society, St. Gallen, Switzerland.

Hoffman, T. C., Montori, V. M., & Del Mar, C. (2014). The Connection Between Evidence-Based Medicine and Shared Decision Making. *Journal of the American Medical Association*, *312*(13), 1295–1296. doi:10.1001/jama.2014.10186 PMID:25268434

Homer, J., & Hirsch, G. (2006). System Dynamics Modeling for Public Health: Background and Opportunities. *American Journal of Public Health*, *96*(3), 452–458. doi:10.2105/AJPH.2005.062059 PMID:16449591

Homer, J., Hirsch, G., Minniti, M., & Pierson, M. (2004). Models for collaboration: How system dynamics helped a community organize cost-effective care for chronic illness. *System Dynamics Review*, *20*(3), 199–222. doi:10.1002dr.295

Johnsson, S., & Lukka, K. (2006). *Doing Interventionist Research in Management Accounting*. Gothenburg, Sweden: Gothenburg Research Institute.

Kannampallil, T. G., Schauer, G. F., Cohen, T., & Patel, V. L. (2011). Considering complexity in healthcare systems. *Journal of Biomedical Informatics*, *44*(6), 943–947. doi:10.1016/j.jbi.2011.06.006 PMID:21763459

Lane, D. C., Monefeldt, C., & Rosenhead, J. V. (2000). Looking in the wrong place for healthcare improvements: A system dynamics study of an accident and emergency department. *The Journal of the Operational Research Society*, *51*(5), 518–531. doi:10.1057/palgrave.jors.2600892

Lattimer, V., Brailsford, S., Turnbull, J., Tarnaras, P., Smith, H., George, S., ... Maslin Prothero, S. (2004). Reviewing emergency care systems I: Insights from system dynamics modelling. *Emergency Medicine Journal*, *21*(6), 685–691. doi:10.1136/emj.2002.003673 PMID:15496694

Loyo, H. K., Batcher, C., Wile, K., Huang, P., Orenstein, D., & Milstein, B. (2013). From model to action: Using system dynamics model of chronic disease risks to align community action. *Health Promotion Practice*, *14*(1), 53–61. doi:10.1177/1524839910390305 PMID:22491443

Marshall, D., Rogers, P., Rohleder, T., & Vanderby, S. (2010). *System Dynamics Modeling: A Decision Support Tool to Improve Care for Hip & Knee Osteoarthritis*. Alberta, Canada: Institute of Health Economics.

Masnick, K., & McDonnell, G. (2010). A model linking clinical workforce skill mix planning to health and healthcare dynamics. *Human Resources for Health*, *8*(1), 11–20. doi:10.1186/1478-4491-8-11 PMID:20433720

Mehrjerdi, Y. Z. (2012). A System Dynamics Approach to Healthcare Cost Control. *International Journal of Industrial Engineering & Production Research*, *23*(3), 175–185.

Merrill, J. A., Deegan, M., Wilson, R. V., Kaushal, R., & Fredericks, K. (2013). A system dynamics evaluation model: Implementation of health information exchange for public health reporting. *Journal of the American Medical Informatics Association*, *20*(1), 131–138. doi:10.1136/amiajnl-2012-001289 PMID:23292910

Patel, V. L., & Cohen, T. (2008). New perspectives on error in critical care. *Current Opinion in Critical Care*, *14*(4), 456–459. doi:10.1097/MCC.0b013e32830634ae PMID:18614912

Pawson, R. (2002). Evidence-based policy. In search of a method (part 1) the promise of 'realist synthesis' (part 2). *Evaluation*, *8*(2), 157–181. doi:10.1177/1358902002008002512

Plesk, P. E., & Wilson, T. (2001). Complexity, leadership and management in healthcare organizations. *British Medical Journal*, *323*, 746–749. doi:10.1136/bmj.323.7315.746 PMID:11576986

Plsek, P. E., & Greenhalgh, T. (2001). The challenge of complexity in healthcare. *British Medical Journal*, *323*, 625–628. doi:10.1136/bmj.323.7313.625 PMID:11557716

Richardson, G. P. (1991). System Dynamics: Simulation for Policy Analysis from a Feedback Perspective. In P. A. Fishwick & P. A. Luker (Eds.), *Qualitative Simulation Modeling and Analysis* (pp. 144–169). New York, NY: Springer-Verlag. doi:10.1007/978-1-4613-9072-5_7

Richardson, G. P. (2011). Reflection on the foundations of system dynamics. *System Dynamics Review*, *27*(3), 219–243. doi:10.1002dr.462

Royston, G., Dost, A., Townshend, J., & Turner, H. (1999). Using system dynamics to help develop and implement policies and programmes in healthcare in England. *System Dynamics Review*, *15*(3), 293–313. doi:10.1002/(SICI)1099-1727(199923)15:3<293::AID-SDR169>3.0.CO;2-1

Rwashana, A. S., Williams, D. W., & Neema, S. (2009). System dynamics approach to immunization healthcare issues in developing countries: A case study in Uganda. *Health Informatics Journal*, *15*(2), 95–107. doi:10.1177/1460458209102971 PMID:19474223

Sackett, D., Richardson, W., Reosenberg, W., & Haynes, R. (1998). *Evidence-based-medicine. How to practice and teach EBM*. London, UK: Churchill Livingstone.

Samuel, C., Gonapa, K., Chaudhary, P. K., & Mishra, A. (2010). Supply chain dynamics in healthcare services. *International Journal of Health Care Quality Assurance*, *23*(7), 631–642. doi:10.1108/09526861011071562 PMID:21125959

Stave, K. A. (2002). Using system dynamics to improve public participation in environmental decisions. *System Dynamics Review*, *18*(2), 139–167. doi:10.1002dr.237

Stave, K. A. (2003). A system dynamics model to facilitate public understanding of water management options in Las Vegas, Nevada. *Journal of Environmental Management*, *67*(4), 303–313. doi:10.1016/S0301-4797(02)00205-0 PMID:12710919

Tuffin, R. (2016). Implications of complexity theory for clinical practice and healthcare organization. *BJA Education*, *16*(10), 349–352. doi:10.1093/bjaed/mkw013

Vennix, J. (2003). *Knowledge Elicitation. Encyclopedia of Life Support Systems (EOLSS). System Dynamics Developed under the Auspices of the UNESCO* (Vol. 2). Paris: Eolss Publishers.

Weaver, W. (1948). Science and complexity. *American Scientist*, *36*(4), 536–544. PMID:18882675

Wittenborn, A. K., Rahmandad, H., Rick, J., & Hosseinichimeh, N. (2015). Depression as a systemic syndrome: Mapping the feedback loops of major depressive disorder. *Psychological Medicine*, *46*(3), 551–562. doi:10.1017/S0033291715002044 PMID:26621339

Wolstenholme, E. (1993). A case study in community care using system thinking. *The Journal of the Operational Research Society*, *44*(9), 925–934. doi:10.1057/jors.1993.160

Wolstenholme, E. (1999). A patient flow perspective of U.K. Health Services: Exploring the case for new "intermediate care" initiatives. *System Dynamics Review*, *15*(3), 253–271. doi:10.1002/(SICI)1099-1727(199923)15:3<253::AID-SDR172>3.0.CO;2-P

Wolstenholme, E., Monk, D., McKelvie, D., & Arnold, G. (2007). Coping but not coping in health and social care: Masking the reality of running organizations beyond safe capacity. *System Dynamics Review*, *23*(4), 371–389. doi:10.1002dr.390

Wolstenholme, E., Monk, D., McKelvie, D., & Smith, G. (2007). Influencing and interpreting health and social care policy in the UK. In Complex decision making. Understanding complex systems (pp. 155-183). Berlin: Springer. doi:10.1007/978-3-540-73665-3_9

Xing, Y., & Dangerfield, B. (2018). Modelling the Sustainability of Mass Tourism in Island Tourist Economies. In M. Kunc (Ed.), *System Dynamics OR Essentials* (pp. 303–327). London, UK: Palgrave Macmillan. doi:10.1057/978-1-349-95257-1_10

Yin, R. K. (2003). *Case Study Research: Design and Methods*. Thousand Oaks, CA: Sage.

ADDITIONAL READING

Barasa, E. W., Molyneux, S., English, M., & Cleary, S. (2017). Hospitals as complex adaptive systems: A case study of factors influencing priority setting practices at the hospital level in Kenya. *Social Science & Medicine*, *174*, 104–112. doi:10.1016/j.socscimed.2016.12.026 PMID:28024239

Dangerfield, B. C. (1999). System dynamics applications to European healthcare issues. *The Journal of the Operational Research Society*, *50*(4), 345–353. doi:10.1057/palgrave.jors.2600729

Lipsitz, L. A. (2012). Understanding Healthcare as a Complex System: The Foundation for Unintended Consequences. *Journal of the American Medical Association*, *308*(3), 243–244. doi:10.1001/jama.2012.7551 PMID:22797640

Marshall, D. A., Burgos-Liz, L., Ijzerman, M. J., Osgood, N. D., Padula, W. D., Higashi, M. K., ... Crown, W. (2015). Applying Dynamic Simulation Modeling Methods in Healthcare Delivery Research -The SIMULATE Checklist: Report of the ISPOR Simulation Modeling Emerging Good Practices Task Force. *Value in Health*, *18*(1), 5–16. doi:10.1016/j.jval.2014.12.001 PMID:25595229

Paina, L., & Peters, D. H. (2012). Understanding pathways for scaling up health services through the lens of complex adaptive systems. *Health Policy and Planning*, *27*(5), 365–373. doi:10.1093/heapol/czr054 PMID:21821667

Trochim, W. M., Cabrera, D. A., Milstein, B., Gallagher, R. S., & Leischow, S. J. (2006). Practical Challenges of Systems Thinking and Modeling in Public Health. *American Journal of Public Health*, *96*(3), 538–546. doi:10.2105/AJPH.2005.066001 PMID:16449581

KEY TERMS AND DEFINITIONS

Causal Loop Diagram: In system dynamics modelling, they are closed causal chains involving relevant variables, whose interactions are responsible for the patterns of behavior taking place within a certain system.

Emergence: Feature of complex systems, meaning that the interactions between system's components lead to unexpected behavioral properties, resulting from system's self-organizational processes.

Flows: State variables' rates of change. In system dynamics, they are represented by pipes, feeding (inflows) or draining (outflows) stock variables.

Interrelatedness: Key property of complex systems defining the level of complexity systems and being the cause of other typical features of complex systems. Interrelatedness means that system components influence each other, so that system complexity increases with the number of its components, the relations between them, and the uniqueness of those relations.

Non-Decomposability: Property of complex systems, according to which the system cannot be fully understood and investigated by just looking at isolated components, but at the interrelations constituting the entire system.

Qualitative System Dynamics Modelling: Representation of dynamic problems by mean of causal loops and stock-and-flow diagrams, with no mathematical formalization of the system dynamics models.

Quantitative System Dynamics Modelling: Representation of dynamic problems by mean of models' mathematical formalization (building of a set of equations representative of decision rules and behavioral relationships), estimations of parameters, testing and calibration. Quantitative SD modelling allows to simulate problematic behaviors and possible scenarios according to different conditions and does not necessarily relate to quantitative researches. Indeed, it is possible to enrich qualitative research design with quantitative SD tools. It is also possible to make statistical analyses on simulated behavior patterns.

Sensitivity to Initial Conditions: A property of complex systems, consisting on the fact that the initial system conditions are able to influence dramatically their behaviors, so that systems with similar structures can witness different behavior patterns (for example exponential growth or decay) due to differences (sometimes slight) in initial parameters.

Stocks: They are the state variables within a certain system. Their level depends on accumulation and depletion processes resulting from the difference between their inflows and outflows.

Uniqueness of Relationships: A factor determining the interrelatedness, and then the complexity, of a system. It means that the complexity of a system does not increase if we just expand its boundaries by mere repetition of relations and components. Then, in order to increase the system's complexity, the new relations need to be unique, original and substantive.

Chapter 6
Modelling Patients' Contribution to Healthcare:
A Dynamic Performance Management Application

ABSTRACT

This chapter proposes an application of simulation modelling to frame the relationships between healthcare, patient organization management, and patient co-created healthcare. For the purpose, it presents a case study within the Italian context, for which it adopts a methodological approach combining performance management and system dynamics. After background information, the chapter introduces the methodology and explains the modelling steps, undertaken assuming the privileged perspective of a patient organization. The model building goes by progressive approximations. A tailored dynamic performance management framework identifies key variables and links within the system. Then a stock-and-flow structure deepens the analysis by depicting processes of accumulation of material, money, and information; a comprehensive loop analysis describes the system's dynamics in terms of interacting feedback structures. Finally, quantitative simulations concerning the mutual development of patient organizations and healthcare allow graphing behavior patterns according to alternative scenarios.

DOI: 10.4018/978-1-7998-2653-8.ch006

BACKGROUND

This chapter investigates patient-aided healthcare through a methodological approach mixing performance management (PM) and system dynamics simulation modelling (SD), to build a dynamic performance management system, or DPMS (Bianchi, 2010; 2012). Recently there was a progressive shift in the definition and measurement of healthcare quality, routed towards patient-centeredness. Patient-centered clinical decisions are the ones capable to reflect informed patients' needs, values, and preferences, in line with a biopsychosocial perspective (Scholl *et al.*, 2014). This concept was associated with improved clinical outcomes, efficiency, and patient satisfaction (Rathert *et al.*, 2013). For these reasons, it is targeted by scholars, policy makers and providers all over the World, striving to find indicators to measure healthcare quality according to patients (Selby & Lipstein, 2014), in the attempt to develop models of 'good healthcare' from the patients' perspective (McCaffrey *et al.*, 2018). Although traditional performance management techniques such as the balanced scorecard (Kaplan & Norton, 1992) in the past have been applied to healthcare organizations (e.g. Inamdar *et al.*, 2000), they fail to capture the multi-dimensionality of healthcare quality. Indeed, such tools are characterized by stativity and are not able to represent the feedback processes involving strategic assets, performance drivers and outcome indicators (Bianchi, 2012).

Quality cannot be assessed just looking at data from administrative or medical records alone, rather requiring direct inputs from patients (Sepucha *et al.*, 2004). The mere implementation of electronic health records is not a patient-centered tool, unless it works for patient-clinician relationships, helping people to know more about their health conditions, and facilitating involvement in their own care (Epstein, & Street, 2011). Then healthcare systems and providers should be modified by mean of a cultural organizational change, from clinician to patient focused (Luxford *et al.*, 2011; Berghout *et al.*, 2015).

In order to deal with these challenges, this chapter pairs performance management with system dynamics (Forrester, 1961; Sterman, 2000), creating synergies between PM's rationale and the potentialities of SD in terms of insight models and simulated policy experiences. Indeed, system dynamics is a flexible methodology, so that it can help to describe multidimensional phenomena such as healthcare, organizational management, learning processes. Thus, the mapping and simulation tools provided by SD can be routed to performance management, or, mirror-like, performance management can be driven, complemented and specified by mean of system dynamics.

TAILORING DYNAMIC PERFORMANCE MANAGEMENT TO PATIENT ORGANIZATIONS

System dynamics is a simulation methodology suitable for investigating any dynamic problem occurring in social, ecologic and/or economic systems, where interdependence, mutual interaction, information feedback, and circular causality take place. SD represents hypothetical causal structures for problematic behaviors, through the following tools:

- Stock-and-flow diagrams (SFD): structures representative of processes of physical, financial or mental accumulation. A SFD is a map made up of three kinds of elements, variously combined: stocks (resource levels at a certain time, graphically portrayed as rectangles); flows (stocks' rates of change, expressed by units per time, represented by pipes); auxiliary (variables helping calculations, also called converters, or playing the role of exogenous parameters or constants. They have circle shapes);
- Causal loop diagrams (CLD): structures portraying feedback circuits interacting each other and determining the system behaviors;
- Computer simulations: SFDs and CLDs are just qualitative and visual representations of quantitative phenomena, that can be formalized through a set of differential equations, linking selected variables of the system and their links. Mathematically SD models are systems of integrals and differential equations, where stocks accumulate their inflows less their outflows, and each flow can be formalized with equations involving other flows, stocks, converters, or estimated parameters or constants. In some cases, the modeler can judge convenient not to represent separately inflows and outflows, and instead to synthesize them in a compact structure, called bi-flow, directly expressive of the net rate of change of a certain stock (Sterman, 2000).

Figure 1 shows an example of stock-and-flow structure illustrating a simplified system characterized by dynamics of resource exploitation driven by movements of population in a certain area. The stock of 'population' is

Figure 1. An example of stock-and-flow diagram

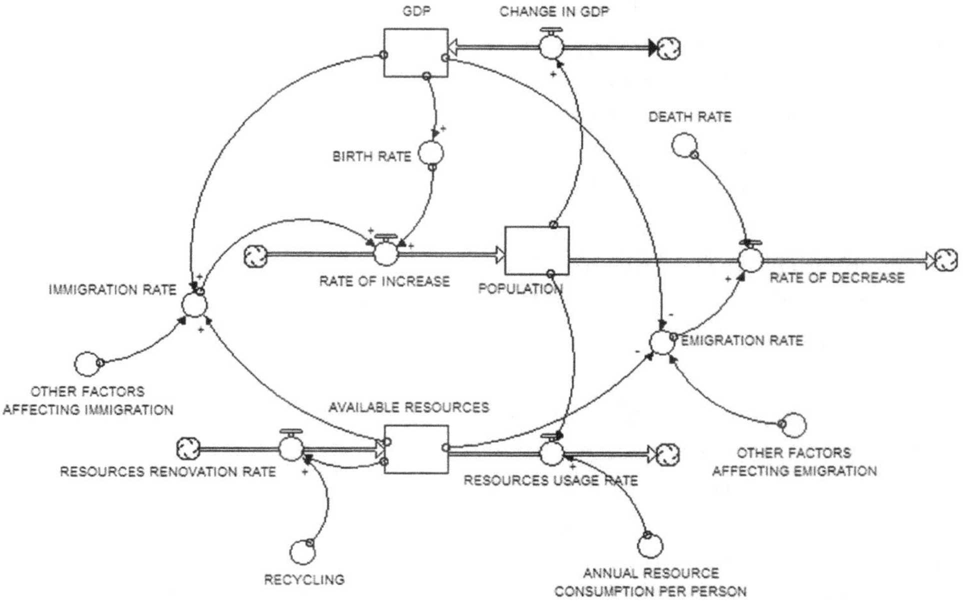

fed by an inflow, the 'rate of increase' and drained by an outflow, the 'rate of decrease'. The population's increase is the sum of two factors: 'birth rate' and 'immigration rate', represented as auxiliary variables. The stock of 'available resources' in the area affects positively the 'immigration rate' and negatively the 'emigration rate'. The accumulation of population in the area, in turn, impacts on the 'resources usage rate', outflowing from the stock of 'available resources'. The population is also linked to GDP, since it is able affect its bi-flow 'change in GDP'. GDP influences positively population, by impacting on 'birth rate' and 'immigration rate'. The model contains exogenous parameters that the author of the chapter decided not to formalize with complex stock-and-flow structures: 'other factors affecting immigration', 'other factors affecting emigration', 'annual resource consumption per person', 'death rate', 'recycling'.

As worth noticing, stocks can determine (directly or by mean of auxiliaries), flows linked to other stocks, creating feedback loops: for example, in the case above 'population' affects the 'resources usage rate', that depletes the stock of 'available resources'. The latter influences both immigration and emigration rates, feeding back into the 'population' stock. Feedback structures can be better pictured by mean of causal loops diagrams, closed causal chains involving relevant variables (Sterman, 2000), for simplicity not distinguishing stock, flow and auxiliaries. CLDs are the manifestation of a key SD principle, i.e. the endogenous point of view (Richardson, 2011), meaning that the internal structure of the model causes behaviors to happen. Figure 2 synthesizes the previous model in a causal loop diagram.

The arrows accompanied by the + sign indicate that there is a positive link between variables: if the first variable increases, *ceteris paribus* (assuming all the other variables constant), the second variable increases; if it decreases, *ceteris paribus* the other variable decreases. A negative link, indicated by the – sign, means that if the independent variable increases, the effect decreases, while if the cause decreases, the effect increases (Sterman, 2000).

Loop R1 is 'reinforcing': this kind of loop operates on the system by emphasizing the initial conditions and triggering virtuous or vicious mechanisms of growth or decay. In general, these loops contain positive links, or an even number of negative links counteracting each other. In the example, a rise in immigration rate provokes population to growth, enhancing GDP, which in turn attracts more immigrants.

The loops indicated by B are 'balancing': they hold an odd number of negative links and, on the contrary, tend to equilibrate or neutralize the initial dynamics. In the example, B1 shows that an increase of population will stimulate the resources usage rate and thereby deplete the stock of available resources. Less resources will result in an increase of emigration and thus in reduction of the population. Moreover, B2 illustrates that the increased

Figure 2. Example of causal loop diagram

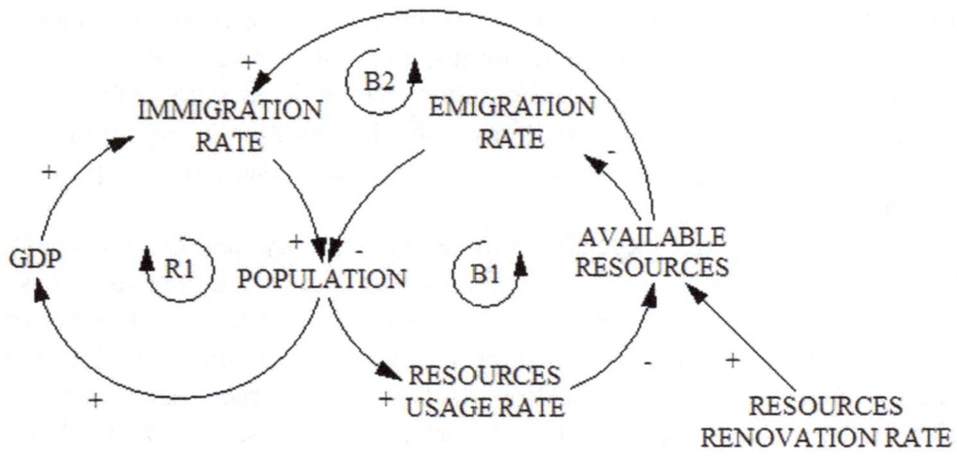

population, provoking a rise in resource consumption, will induce immigration to reduce, thereby draining the level of population.

The 'dynamic performance management' approach (Bianchi, 2010; 2012) proposed in this chapter requires two contemporary and iterative processes. On the one hand, that the guiding principles of PM are enclosed in the SD modelling: then the model will depict a performance-driven causal tissue, willing to identify key-performance indicators and the factors affecting them. On the other side, it requires that the selection of variables being part of the performance system takes place in consideration of their possible translation into SD building blocks: stock, flows, auxiliaries and feedbacks. Figure 3 represents a general framework to conduct this kind of analysis.

The framework above illustrates that a DPMS is made of three components: strategic resources, performance drivers and end-results; and juxtaposes them to SD blocks, respectively stocks, auxiliaries and flows. Then strategic resources are sketched through stocks because the system can accumulate or deplete them through external acquisitions/transfers, or internal building/depletion. Furthermore, they are able to influence the acquisition of other resources and the system's capacity to move towards its goals. Performance drivers, modelled as auxiliary variables, are critical success factors able to influence the end-results. The latter, represented by flows, are socio-economic results

Figure 3. Dynamic performance management framework (Bianchi, 2010)

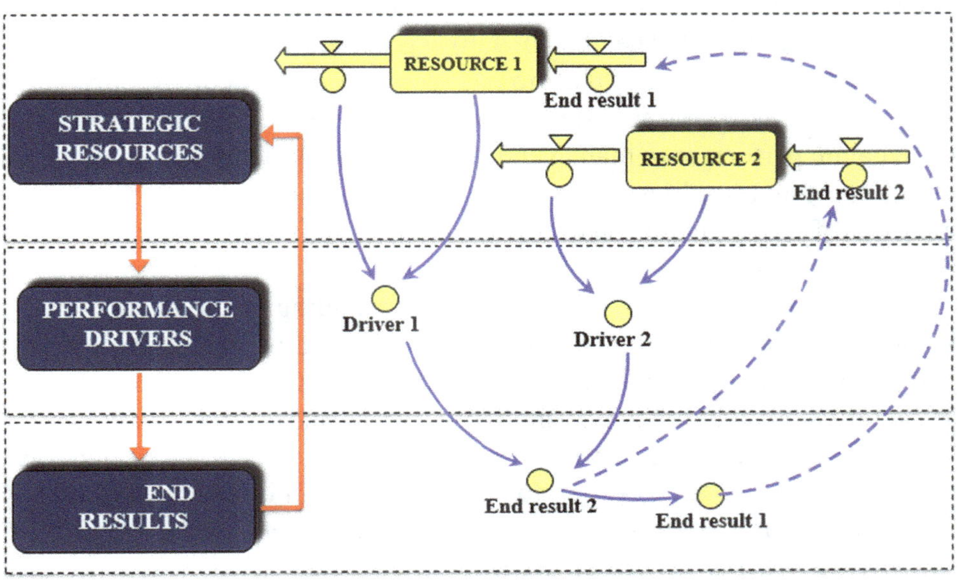

occurring in a certain period, able to affect the processes of accumulation/ depletion of the strategic resources over the time.

MODEL BUILDING ACTIVITIES

The model of patient organization-aided healthcare proposed in this chapter combines two complementary perspectives of patient contribution to healthcare. The first refers to patient representative organizations, able to operate in grey areas where public service is lacking, or to 'educate' individual patients (with the aim to improve their healthcare literacy), and physicians (to enhance their communication skills), this way corroborating healthcare co-creative processes. According to this first perspective, the model focuses two main streams of patient organizations' contributions: through education (to physicians and to peers) and through operational support to healthcare. The second perspective considers individual patients whose aggregated preferences and potentially virtuous behaviors (eventually triggered/enhanced by patient organizations) co-create value for themselves and for the community.

For the purpose of the research, it was decided to study the case of a patient organization targeting a specific disease, the thyroid cancer, considered chronic since it requires surgical treatment, periodical follow-ups to surveille recidivisms, as well as lifelong substitutive therapies.

A four-phase process, proceeding by gradual approximation, lead to the model's conceptualization and formalization. The first phase enclosed the mapping of patient-aided healthcare delivery macro-processes. In the second phase, model boundaries and partitions (sectors) were decided. The third stage consisted on the explosion of such sketches into a more complex framework, the dynamic performance management system. The last step was the system dynamics' model building *strictu sensu*, aimed at formalizing variables' links, processes of accumulation, feedback mechanisms, differential equations, and simulated scenario analyses.

Each step, in pace with the author's understanding of the phenomenon, provided a more analytical version of the model iteratively built in previous phases: for this reason, in the study the terms 'model', and 'framework' can be used either to identify the final modelling output and the intermediate ones. Inputs to the model building were relevant literature and empirical findings. In particular, the author took part to a one-year project involving, among the others, an Italian patient's organization (period January-December 2014). The 'mental models' of key actors were investigated through unstructured and semi-structured interviews to physicians working at public hospitals and to patient organizations' members, and the administration of questionnaires to patients.

First Step: Sketching Patient-Aided Healthcare Delivery Value Chain

The first modelling step was a preliminary map of healthcare provision, aiming to identify macro-processes, key actors taking part to them and their specific contribution to the complex final product 'patient health'. The concept of product is not limited to the final product for the 'external client', i.e. health for patients, but also to 'intermediate products' which the 'internal clients', actors within the value chain, can benefit. Backward from the final product, it was re-constructed a synthetic system of intermediate products resulting from processes performed by several actors of a Local Healthcare Authority. Figure 4 portrays the performance cycle regarding the thyroid cancer management and other related pathologies in an endemic area.

The performance cycle starts with the General Practitioner activity, whose intermediate product consists of 'pathology suspects'. Then, patients are directed to the outpatient clinic, which will provide 'diagnoses' as intermediate product. Afterwards, the hospital will provide 'surgeries' for the patients needing them, and again, the outpatient clinic will bring 'follow-ups' as required by protocols.

A relevant portion of the model is devoted to the outpatient clinic, since the case study targets the activities of a patients' organization operating in that theatre. The framework follows both an inter-institutional and value co-creative perspective. Indeed, the patient plays a double role as consumer and individual co-creator, in this activity boosted by a patients' organization. In detail, the patient's perspective helps the outpatient clinic to produce 'diagnoses' and contributes to his/her own health by mean of 'fulfilled therapy requirements'. The patients' organization cooperates with patients and clinicians in the diagnostic and following-up phases, bringing educational and operational (especially in the administrative sphere) support to patients and clinicians.

Second Step: Identifying Key Model Sectors

Based on the previous framework, this stage implied decisions about boundaries and partitions of the model. In particular, the model was articulated into three

Figure 4. Value chain of patient-aided healthcare

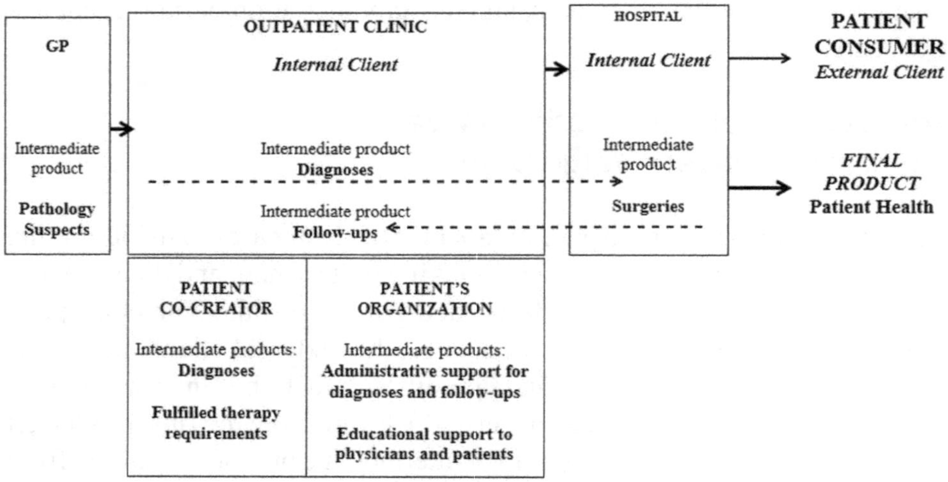

sectors (figure 5), enclosing variables and links characterized by process homogeneity. The first sector is 'delivery of healthcare', whose focus was the illustration of the diagnostic-therapeutic path. Following the inter-institutional perspective stated above, it was decided to model the healthcare delivery as a unique process, despite several actors' participation. The second sector is 'patient organization's management', aiming to depict the core activities of the investigated patients' organization, their impacts on the other sectors and the relevant financial dynamics. The third sector is devoted to 'patient co-created healthcare'. Such partition of the model has the purpose to depict patients-physicians' interactions, and their effects on diagnostic-therapeutic processes and on patients' capacity to adhere to recommended therapies. In this regard, the educational role of the patients' organization needs highlight.

Third Step: Framing Dynamic Performance Management System

Keeping in mind the model sectors introduced in step 2 and the value chain sketched in step 1, the author progressively collected inputs from literature and empirical findings about key-variables involved in patient-aided healthcare. This phase allowed hypothesizing the dynamic performance management system resulting from the interaction of strategic resources, performance drivers and end-results. The output of the process is the model in figure 6.

Figure 5. Model sectors and their focus

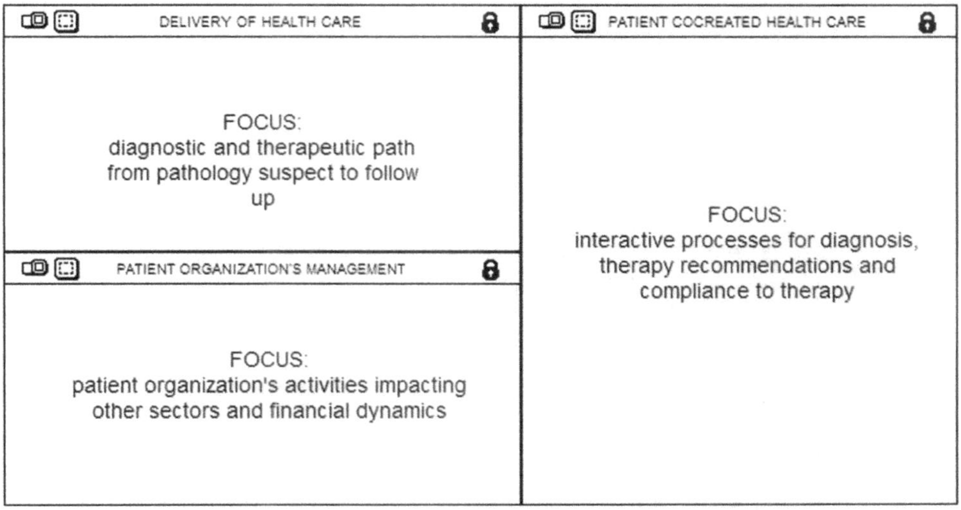

This modelling phase started with the identification, for each sector, of key strategic resources (SD stocks), whose importance lays in their ability to influence performance drivers and thereby end-results. The selected variables are both tangible (patient organization's cumulated earnings, paid volunteers) and intangible (e.g. perceived quality of healthcare, healthcare literacy).

The strategic resources included in the sector 'delivery of healthcare' are basically patients' stocks. As patients proceed in the diagnostic-therapeutic path, several stocks are respectively fed and drained by in- and outflows: waiting lists (for diagnosis and for follow-up), stocks of 'outpatients', 'patients needing surgery', and 'people needing follow-up'.

Among the strategic resources enclosed in the sector 'patient organization's management':

- 'cumulated patient members': this stock accumulates the annual rate of enrolment to the patients' organization. It contains not just people affected by the disease, but it may include family members, caregivers, philanthropists and sympathizers;
- 'patient organization's cumulated earning': as operating in the third sector, patients' organization does not distribute earnings to its members and rather accumulates them for allocation on investments. Given the shortage of public and industry funds, on an annual basis

Figure 6. Dynamic performance management framework tailored to patient-aided healthcare

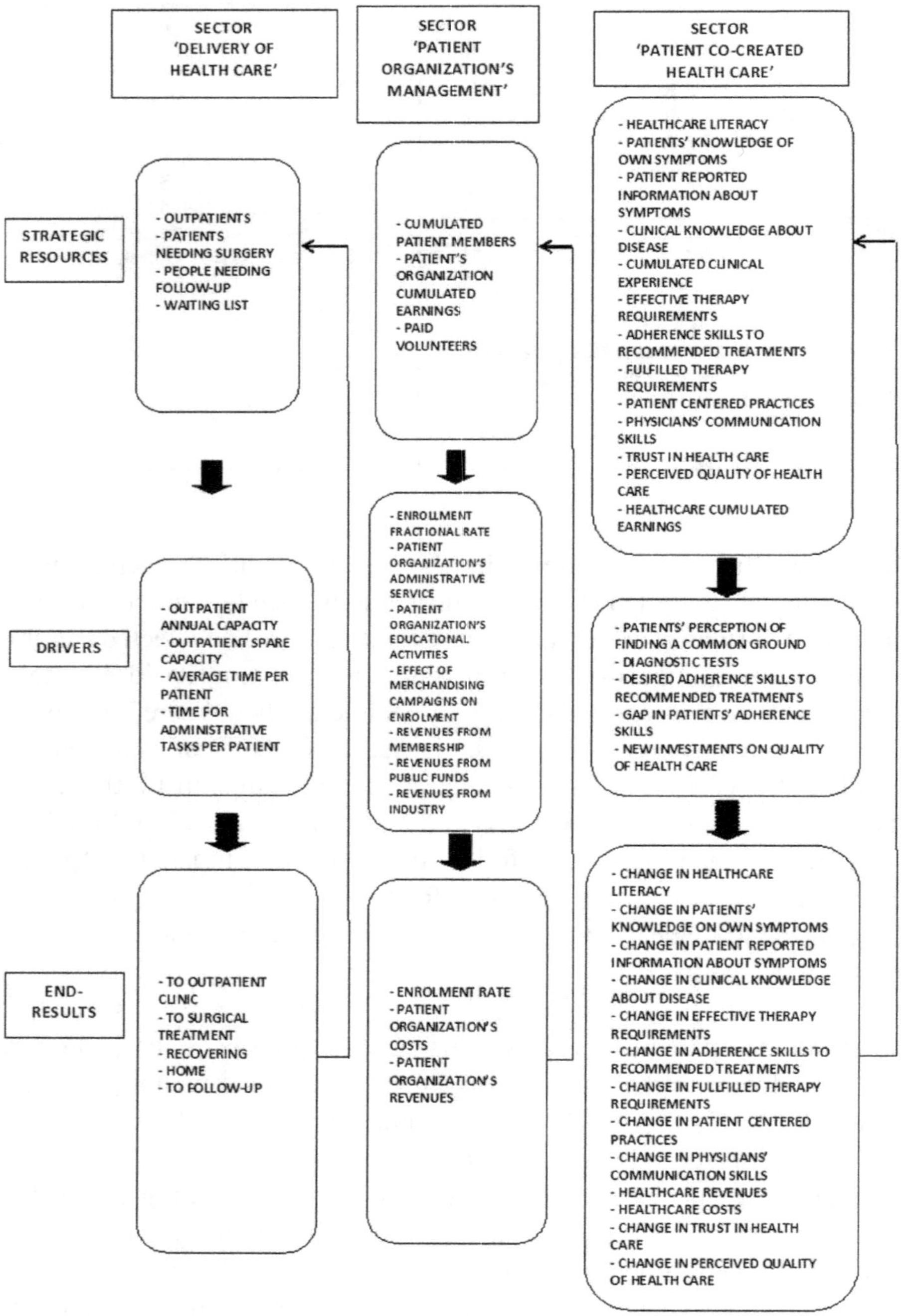

the organization strives to balance costs and revenues, and, even when revenues overcome costs, the earnings are re-invested;

- 'paid volunteers': this represents the number of volunteers bringing a relevant amount of their time and efforts to the organization's initiatives. It is important to distinguish them from the case of non-paid volunteers, who work with no compensation because they are not involved on a daily basis (just devoting to the patients' organization a couple of hours per week or every second week). On the contrary, paid volunteers dedicate plenty of time to volunteering, they produce added value, so that they mean their action within the organization as a work, requiring a compensation. However, their nature remains voluntary, since the average compensation per volunteer (about 300 euro per month) is not aligned to salary standard, rather constituting a repayment for fuel costs or for public transport.

Finally, the sector of 'patient co-created healthcare' puts together and builds on two qualitative models from literature. The first, developed by Elg and colleagues (2012), illustrates processes of learning and co-creation in the healthcare sector. The second model provides a feedback-based application of patient-centeredness in the context of chronic illnesses (Shippee *et al.*, 2012). In the latter, health outcomes result from the balance between patient workload required to comply with therapies and patient capacity to address such demand. Considering these inputs, the model includes many 'mental stocks', i.e. stocks representing soft variables. So far, the only non-mental stock identified is the 'healthcare cumulated earnings', chosen because patient centered practices (Luxford *et al.*, 2011), by conducting to better diagnostic processes, reduce the number of diagnostic tests (Bertakis & Azari, 2011; Kim *et al.* 2017), thereby diminishing costs and, *ceteris paribus*, increasing cumulated earnings. Given the case study of public health, earnings are not distributed and tend to be reinvested to improve quality of healthcare services.

The soft strategic variables are:

- 'Healthcare literacy': it can trigger quality of healthcare (Altin & Stock, 2015; Mc Lean *et al.*, 2019), both in terms of patient support to diagnosis and to ability to comply with medical recommendations;
- 'Patient knowledge on own symptoms': this variable accumulates inputs from media, experience, word-of-mouth (WOM), and any other source able to improve the patients' level of information about their condition. Patients, in particular the chronic ones, can be considered

experts of their own status, thus their contribution to healthcare cannot be underestimate (Kane *et al.*, 2015; Tobiano *et al.*, 2018);

- 'Clinical knowledge about disease': stock accumulating the information progressively acquired by physicians about the clinical cases under investigation. This stock is also determined by shared information between patients and clinicians, progressively driving to a shared decision-making (Verwijmeren & Grootens, 2018);
- 'Cumulated clinical experience': this stock refers to the physicians' comprehensive experience, able to drive continuous learning by doing, and improvement in the diagnostic-therapeutic processes;
- 'Effective therapy requirements': this is a variable accumulating the physicians' recommendations leading to effective patients' health;
- 'Fulfilled therapy requirements': stock of therapy items followed by patients in light of another stock, the 'adherence skills to recommended treatments', representing the patients' ability to cope with therapy requirements. Especially for chronic diseases, the effectiveness of medical interventions is undermined by lacks in this sphere (Shippee *et al.*, 2012);
- 'Patient-centered practices': patient-centered healthcare leads to quality, accessibility, efficiency and effectiveness. In this model, the actual level of patient-centered practices (Santana *et al.* 2017), taking place within the process of healthcare provision, impacts positively on the 'clinical knowledge about disease' (introduced above) and at the same time reduces the costs for 'diagnostic tests'. For example, collection routines of patient feedbacks after healthcare episodes (e.g. low-cost online patient-centered care surveys), could be used by physicians to understand what went right/wrong from the perspective of the patients and to suggest opportunities for improvement (Davis *et al.*, 2005);
- Variables related to communication, quality and trust: in the model, despite the patients' skill development, dynamics of 'physicians communication skills' are important vehicles towards patient compliance to care. The model also portrays a multi-dimensional causal tissue of the 'perceived quality of healthcare'. This stock affects another strategic variable, 'trust in healthcare', by mean of its inflow. Indeed, patients' trust in healthcare providers may affect their satisfaction and health outcomes (Fiscella *et al.*, 2004), and its accumulation is considered as a predictor of patient engagement (Ford-Gilboe *et al.*, 2018), and as an enhancer of patient capabilities (Terry &

Kayes, 2019). Furthermore, trusting patients are more likely to disclose important information (Sarango *et al.*, 2018). It is also recognized the importance to fill their information gap, as a mean ensuring health quality (Sepucha *et al.*, 2004).

After identification of strategic resources, it was selected a set of performance drivers (SD auxiliary variables), representing the system's capacity to pursue its objectives through critical success factors. For the sector 'delivery of healthcare', relevant drivers are 'outpatient annual capacity' and 'outpatient spare capacity': the 'outpatient spare capacity' regulates the access of patients into the outpatient clinic. It depends on the 'outpatients' (i.e. capacity in use) and on the 'annual capacity of the outpatient clinic' (potential capacity). The annual capacity can be calculated by considering the physicians as a scarce resource. By estimating the 'average time per patient' as a sum of times for medical and administrative tasks, the case study reveals that physicians dedicate half of the time to non-medical tasks because of administrative and nursing personnel's shortages. They regulate access queueing, patient booking, pre-registration and registration. Furthermore, a relevant bottleneck exists because after the start of the visit, patients need to move to an administrative office to pay the fee to access the public healthcare service. Then the doctor, instead of waiting for their return, will start another visit or continue a visit previously started to people that have already paid their due. Such breaks interrupt the patient-doctor flows of information exchanges, make waiting times longer and do the same with the 'average time per patient'. Then the model shows how the patients' organization can intervene by reducing the 'time for administrative tasks per patient', thereby freeing up new outpatient capacity.

In the 'patient organization's management' sector, the most important performance drivers are:

- The 'enrolment fractional rate': it is the fraction of patients, families, caregivers, philanthropists and sympathizers that enroll on an annual basis. In turn, it is affected by other drivers, each of them representing the impact of the patient organization's streams of activity on people's attitude to sustain it. In particular, the case study's organization works in three strategic areas: administrative support within the outpatient clinic, education to patients and physicians, and merchandising campaigns (carried on collecting donations versus small gadgets bought at discounted prices for sponsorships). Then, among the performance drivers there are: 'patient organizations' administrative service', 'patient organizations' educational activities', and 'effect of merchandising campaigns on enrolment';

- 'Revenues from public funds' and 'from industry': the merchandising campaigns were modelled as only representing about the 20% of the organizational budget, whilst the core funding sources are public funding and industry. Their amount was hypothesized proportional to the patient members' basis, so the patients' organization must pursue a consistent enrolment rate in order to maintain external funding sources.
- In the sector of 'patient co-created healthcare' few identified drivers are technical ('diagnostic tests') or financial ('new investments on quality of healthcare'), whilst the majority is immaterial. The 'patient perception of finding a common ground' (with doctors), retrieved from literature (Stewart *et al.*, 2000), is strictly related to patient-centered practices and perceived quality of the healthcare. Other drivers are the 'desired skills to recommended treatment' and the 'gap in adherence skills', occurring by comparing desired and actual patient skills.
- Finally, the framework highlights end-results registered by the relevant system in a certain timeframe, the SD flows, able to feed back into the processes of strategic resources' accumulation/depletion. The most relevant end-results of the model are described below:
- In the sector of 'delivery of healthcare', the patients' routes through the diagnostic-therapeutic path are tracked by flow of patients at different stages of care. Most of the times, the outflow from a certain stock is the inflow of another one. For example, patients 'to outpatient clinic' represent an outflow from 'waiting list' and an inflow to the 'outpatients' stock;
- In the sector of 'patient organization's management', key end-results are the annual 'enrolment rate' and the financial results (patient organization's costs and revenues);
- In the sector of 'patient co-created healthcare', beside healthcare costs and revenues, the majority of end-results consists on the changes of the strategic variables over the time, for example, 'change in healthcare literacy', 'change in patient knowledge on own symptoms' and 'change in adherence skills to recommended treatments'.

Fourth Step: Designing a System Dynamics Model

The dynamic performance management framework presented above was translated into a SD model: the stock notation was used to represent the strategic resources, able to impact on performance drivers (calculating variables) thereby affecting the end-results (flows), that feed back into the stocks.

The comprehensive conceptual scheme in figure 7 synthesizes how the sector 'patient organization's management' intermediates between the other two. For each sector it was chosen a representative stock: 'outpatients', 'cumulated patient members' and 'perceived quality of healthcare'. Two contributions of the patient organization's sector to the other ones are shown: administrative support, mainly devoted to 'delivery of healthcare', and educational support, directed to the 'patient co-created healthcare'. Then the model is in line with the contemporary consciousness about patients' role. For long time excluded from healthcare decisional processes, they are called to share responsibilities with physicians about medical paths. This fact leads to new educational needs, providing patients with healthcare literacy and making them aware of the essential role they play (Barry & Edgman-Levitan, 2012). On the other side, the shift from a professional to a patient-centered healthcare (Fiorio *et al.*, 2018; Prag *et al.*, 2017), requires filling communication gaps between patients and doctors (McCabe & Healey, 2018).

The next three figures show the complete stock-and-flow structure of each sector. The delivery of healthcare (figure 8) is made of four stocks, representing the stages of healthcare provision identified above. The input to the entire model is the inflow 'people needing treatment', depending on the variables 'waiting time before access' and 'GP referrals', in turn determined by the 'population' in the area and the 'morbidity incidence rate'. People needing treatment accumulate into the stock 'waiting list', drained by the outflow 'to outpatient clinic', that converges as an inflow to the stock 'outpatients'. The flow 'to outpatient clinic' represents the movement of people being visited and it is affected by the 'outpatient spare capacity', calculated as difference between the 'outpatient annual capacity' (current capacity) and 'outpatients' (capacity in use).

The 'annual outpatient capacity' is set in terms of outpatients that could be visited yearly according to available scarce resources, i.e. people and time. It is calculated by multiplying the number of 'physicians' and the 'working hours per physician per year' and dividing the result for the 'average time per patient'. The latter is the sum of times for medical and administrative

Figure 7. Synthetic view of the model: sectors, key stocks and their interrelationships

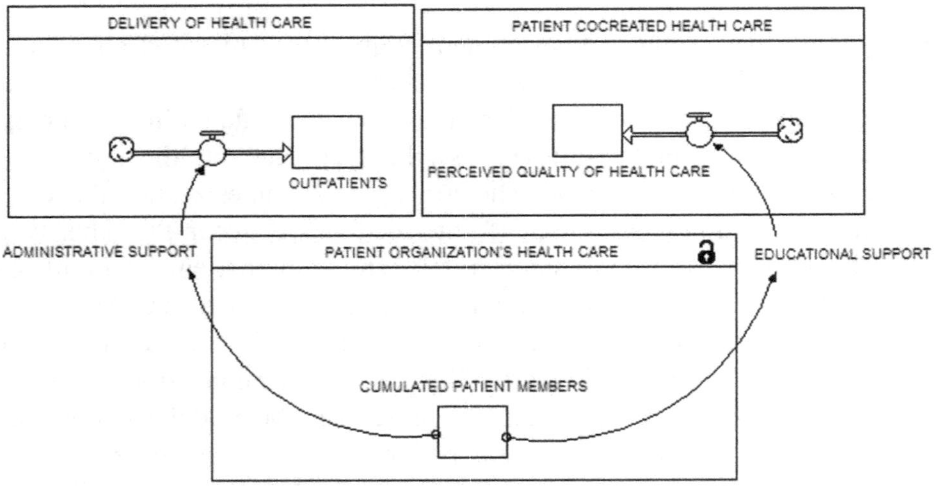

tasks. In the case study, due to administrative personnel's shortage, doctors must spend one portion of the working time by doing administrative rather than medical tasks. Since the administrative tasks are relatively simple, not requiring high professionalization (e.g. welcoming people, registering them, regulating queues) they can be fulfilled by patient organization's volunteers. Then the 'time for administrative tasks per patient' has a policy potential, because through the 'patient organization's administrative service', it is possible to free up medical capacity and thereby to increase the 'annual outpatient capacity'.

After the visit, people flow out from the 'outpatients' stock and two routes are possible: one 'to surgical treatment', regulated by the annual 'fraction (of patients) needing surgery' and one going 'home', whose fraction is the complement to 1 of the 'fraction needing surgery'. After operation, people will need follow-up every year ('follow up time' set at value 1), so the flow 'to follow-up' will progressively accumulate into the 'waiting list', creating new demand for outpatient services.

In the sector 'Patient organization's management' (figure 9), the stock of 'cumulated patient members' accumulates the 'enrolment rate' (people per year), resulting from the multiplication of 'outpatients' and 'enrolment fractional rate' (fraction of people per year). This comes from the combination of 'effect of merchandising campaigns on enrolment' and 'effect of service quality improvement on enrolment'. The first effect can be considered as a

Figure 8. Delivery of healthcare: stock-and-flow structure

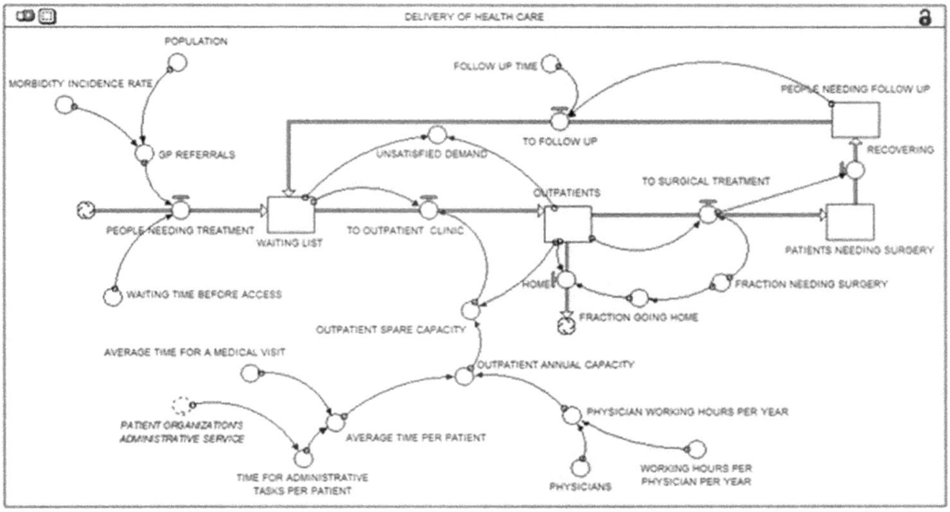

word-of-mouth from brand ambassadors, whilst the second one is due to perceived quality improvements driven by activities of patient organizations: 'patient organization's educational activities' and 'patient organization's administrative service' within the outpatient clinic.

From the stock of 'cumulated patient members' descends three kinds of revenues: 'revenues from public funds', 'revenues from industry' and 'revenues from membership' according to the annual association fee. Together with the 'revenues from merchandising', they sum up in the flow of 'patient organization revenues', and thus in the stock of 'patient organization's cumulated earnings', from which the 'patient organization's costs' flow out.

From the stock of 'cumulated patient members' descends three kinds of revenues: 'revenues from public funds', 'revenues from industry' and 'revenues from membership' according to the annual association fee. Such revenues, together with the 'revenues from merchandising', sum in the flow of 'patient organization's revenues', converging into the stock of 'patient organization's cumulated earnings', from which the 'patient organization's costs' flow out.

The costs' structure highlights 'compensation to paid volunteers' (multiplication of stock 'paid volunteers' and 'average compensation per volunteer'), and merchandising costs as key 'operating variable costs', whilst the remaining cost types (computers, mobile phones, electric bills, rent) are inserted into 'other costs'. The cumulated earnings consent to hire 'paid volunteers',

Figure 9. Patient organization's management: stock-and-flow structure

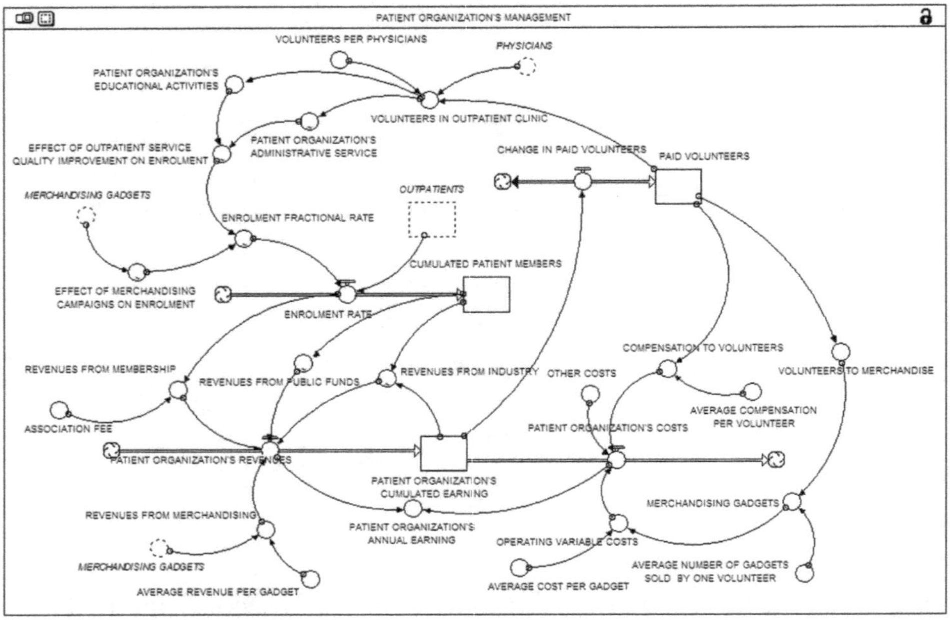

that can be employed alternatively into administrative and educational tasks, respectively within the outpatient clinic or into merchandising campaigns. The number of 'merchandising gadgets' (to be purchased and re-sold) is determined by the allocation of paid volunteers to merchandising activities, by considering the 'average number of gadgets sold by one volunteer'.

Figure 10 portrays the stock-and-flow structure of the sector 'patient co-created healthcare'. On the left side, the stock of 'perceived quality of healthcare' is the result of the dynamics occurring in the bi-flow 'change in perceived quality of healthcare', which is function of three variables: the 'effective quality of healthcare', the 'patient perception of finding a common ground' with physicians, and the stock of 'fulfilled therapy requirements'. From the 'perceived quality of healthcare' departs a cascade of stocks and flows. Perceived quality affects 'trust in healthcare', the latter influences 'patient reported information about symptoms' and patient 'propensity to adhere' to recommended treatments. The model distinguishes the patients' attitude towards adherence to doctors' recommendation and the effective put in practice of such backlog. In order to increase the stock of 'fulfilled therapy requirements', there are necessary 'adherence skills to recommended treatment', that depend on 'propensity to adhere' and on 'healthcare literacy'. The bi-flow 'change in fulfilled therapy requirements' depends on the 'gap in patient adherence skills', obtained by difference between 'desired adherence skills to recommended treatments' and actual adherence skills.

'Healthcare literacy' is related to 'patient knowledge on own symptoms' and 'patient organization's educational activities', this last variable being a connector between this sector and the one of 'patient organization's management'. Many sources of information affect the 'change in patient knowledge on own symptoms': knowledge from previous healthcare experiences, media (traditional or digital), word-of-mouth and 'clinical knowledge about disease'. The latter represents an informative flow to patients from the physicians taking in charge their care. The 'patient knowledge of own symptoms', together with 'trust in healthcare' and 'healthcare literacy', cause the stock of 'patient reported information about symptoms' to change. This is because it may happen that patients, although realizing to feel certain health conditions, are not aware of their relevance as possible symptoms, or are not able to report about their physical sensations because of lack in healthcare literacy. Patient reported symptoms cause the 'patient-centered practices' to accumulate, and this has a depletive effect on 'diagnostic tests' and thereby on 'healthcare costs'. Such savings are destined to 'new investment of quality healthcare', contributing to the 'effective quality of healthcare'. Patient-centered practices, together with diagnostic tests and patient-reported

Figure 10. Patient co-created healthcare: stock-and-flow structure

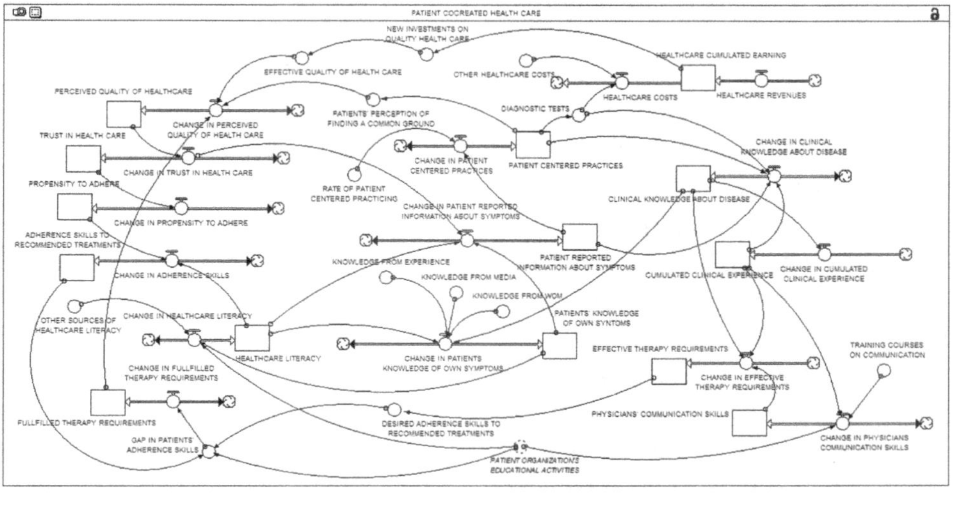

information about symptoms, determine the change of the stock of 'clinical knowledge about disease', and by this way physicians progressively learn by experience, so that their 'cumulated clinical experience' increases over the time.

Clinical knowledge about disease, cumulated clinical experience and 'physicians' communication skills' are determinants of the 'change in effective therapy requirements'. This part of the model structure reflects the call for a combination of evidence-based medicine and shared decision making. Indeed, according to Hoffman *et al.* (2014), evidence-based medicine has the patient as a starting and ending point. Doctors proceed by finding evidences about the cases and integrate their inferences with their expertise. Then they should take a clinical decision incorporating patient's values, preferences and circumstances. The use of the adjective 'effective' is not casual and emphasizes the central role of communication skills for the effectiveness of therapy recommendation. Indeed, for a good medical doctor it is not important just clinical knowledge able to convey suitable prescriptions, but also the ability to communicate such prescriptions. Physicians' communication skills depend on the experience, but according to literature, they are normally underdeveloped and there is a call for their inclusion into medical training programs (McCabe & Healey, 2018). In this regard, 'patient organization's educational activities' can contribute to the enhancement of physicians' communication skills.

MODEL ANALYSIS

Loop Analysis

A system dynamics model has the merit to capture a certain phenomenon as a network of feedbacks including stock, flows and auxiliary variables. The feedback structure of the model and its core dynamics can be synthesized and analyzed through comprehensive causal loops diagrams (CLDs). They are close cause-and-effect chains not distinguishing stocks, flows and auxiliaries, and isolating relevant variables from the ones belonging to the stock-and-flow structure.

In order to pursue clarity of exposition, it was decided to articulate the model's loop analysis in two parts: one combining patient organization and outpatient clinic's dynamics (CLD in figure 11), and one focusing patient co-created healthcare processes (CLD in figure 12). However, these two major loops are meant to be viewed as complementary, and each of them is the result of the interaction of many minor loops.

The CLD in figure 11 contains 13 loops, 11 of them are reinforcing (denoted by an R followed by a number) and 2 balancing (B followed by numbers). In order to shed light into the complexity of such net of relations, these loops can be grouped in three sub-categories according to homogenous criteria:

- Loops regarding the mutual development dynamics of outpatient clinic and patients' organization;
- Loops regarding the enrolment dynamics of patients' organization;
- Loops regarding patient organization's financial performances.

Figure 11. Causal loop diagram integrating sectors of 'delivery of healthcare' and 'patient organization's management'

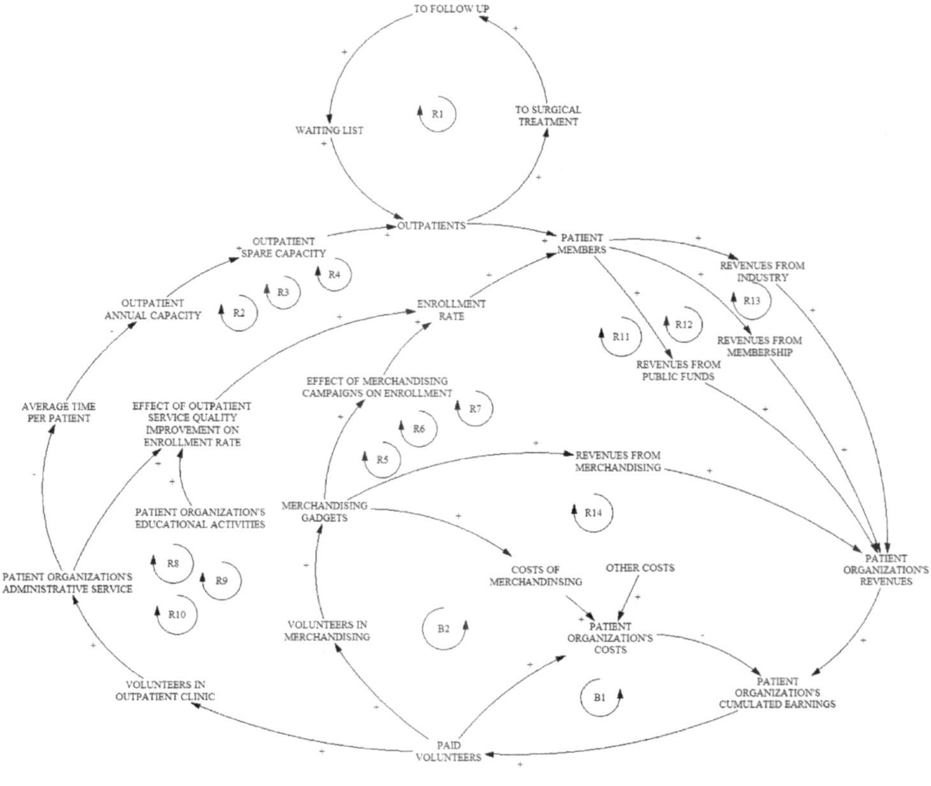

The first group of loops isolates mutually reinforcing dynamics of the outpatient clinic and the patients' organization. It is composed by four reinforcing loops, from R1 to R4, whose chains are reported in table 1. Loop R1 shows how outpatients' dynamics are physiologically driven by the characteristics of the diagnostic and therapeutic path. More people in waiting list, *ceteris paribus*, increase the outpatients, an increase of which will cause people undergoing to surgical treatments to raise and, according to guidelines, to be followed up. A rise in the follow-up activity has a stimulating effect on the demand for outpatient services, so that the circuit restarts and will have the tendency to reinforce itself. The loop can also work creating decay dynamics, i.e. a decrease in the waiting list or in any of the variables of the chain will have a diminishing domino effect.

Loops R2, R3 and R4 illustrate how patient organization's enlargement (in terms of membership), has a positive effect on 'outpatients', and then on the satisfied demand of healthcare. The growth of patient members is driven by three streams of financial resources (public funds, membership fees and industry funds), that can be allocated to administrative services brought by volunteers to the outpatient clinic. This figure, supporting healthcare in the administrative sphere, has a positive effect on the outpatient capacity, depending on available funds to compensate paid volunteers which collaborate with physicians. In R2, an increase of volunteers in the outpatient clinic causes a reduction in the 'average time per patient', thus freeing up new 'outpatient annual capacity', 'outpatient spare capacity' and 'outpatients'. More 'outpatients' means more 'patient members', a rise of 'revenues from public funds' (since in the model they are aligned to the organizational members), and thus more paid volunteers to allocate to outpatient clinic.

On the other way around, the loop can work unfavourably, so that a reduction in the number of volunteers can have a depleting cascade effect. Similar dynamics can be observed in loop R3 and R4: the structure of these loops is identical to R1, excepted for the variables representing the funding sources, that instead of public funds, are 'revenues from membership' and 'revenues from industry'.

The second group of loops isolates the enrolment dynamics within the patient organization. The development of the member basis is trained by three types of financial resources (revenues from public funds, from membership and from industry), to be partially used to compensate 'paid volunteers', that can either be allocated to administrative tasks in the outpatient clinic or to merchandising activities. From the possible combinations of such funding

Table 1. Mutual development of outpatient clinic and patient organization: causal loops

LOOP	VARIABLES
R1.	Waiting list → Outpatients → To surgical treatment → To follow up
R2.	Average time per patient → Outpatient annual capacity → Outpatient spare capacity → Outpatients → Patient members → Revenues from public funds → Patient organization's revenues → Patient organization's cumulated earnings → Paid volunteers → Volunteers in outpatient clinic → Patient organization's administrative service capacity
R3.	Outpatients → Patient members → Revenues from membership → Patient organization's revenues → Patient organization's cumulated earnings → Paid volunteers → Volunteers in outpatient clinic → Patient organization's administrative service → Average time per patient → Outpatient annual capacity → Outpatient spare capacity
R4.	Outpatients → Patient members → Revenues from industry → Patient organization's revenues → Patient organization's cumulated earnings → Paid volunteers → Volunteers in outpatient clinic → Patient organization's administrative service → Average time per patient → Outpatient annual capacity → Outpatient spare capacity

and allocative possibilities descend six reinforcing loops, from R5 to R10, whose complete variable chains are reported in table 2.

Loop R5 shows how enrolment rate can be affected by public funds and merchandising campaigns. An increment of 'patient members' causes the 'revenues from public funds' to increase and so for the overall 'patient organization revenues' and earnings. This allows to hire more 'paid volunteers' and, *ceteris paribus*, to devote more 'volunteers in merchandising', that will sell more gadgets and, by being ambassadors of the patient organization's brand, have a boosting effect on the enrolment rate. Loops R6 and R7 depict similar dynamics, with the difference that their circuits use different funding sources to merchandising allocation.

Loop 8 highlights changes in the enrolment rate due to revenues from public funds and patient organization's administrative support in the outpatient clinic. More patient organization's members attract public funds, thereby increasing revenues and earnings. This fact allows the hiring of more paid volunteers, to be allocated to outpatient clinic, contributing to outpatient service quality and driving new enrolments. Loops 9 and 10 illustrate similar dynamics, respectively fed by revenues from membership and from industry.

The third group of loops isolates some financial movements taking place within the patient organization. Their notations, descriptions and variable chains are presented in table 3. Loop 11 shows the effect of an increase of paid volunteers and their allocation on merchandising activities. Indeed, an augment of 'paid volunteers' consents to devote more 'volunteers in merchandising', and then to sell more gadgets. The latter will provoke an

Table 2. Development dynamics of patient organization: causal loops

LOOP	VARIABLES
R5.	Patient members → Revenues from public funds → Patient organization's revenues → Patient organization's cumulated earnings → Paid volunteers → Volunteers in merchandising → Merchandising gadgets → Effect of merchandising campaigns on enrolment → Enrolment rate
R6.	Patient members → Revenues from membership → Patient organization's revenues → Patient organizations' cumulated earnings → Paid volunteers → Volunteers in merchandising → Merchandising gadgets → Effect of merchandising campaigns on enrolment → Enrolment rate
R7.	Patient members → Revenues from industry → Patient organization's revenues → Patient organization's cumulated earnings → Paid volunteers → Volunteers in merchandising → Merchandising gadgets → Effect of merchandising campaigns on enrolment → Enrolment rate
R8.	Patient members → Revenues from public funds → Patient organization's revenues → Patient organization's cumulated earnings → Paid volunteers → Volunteers in outpatient clinic → Patient organization's administrative service → Effect of outpatient service quality improvement on enrolment rate → Enrolment rate
R9.	Patient members → Revenues from membership → Patient organization's revenues → Patient organization's cumulated earnings → Paid volunteers → Volunteers in outpatient clinic → Patient organization's administrative service → Effect of outpatient service quality improvement on enrolment rate → Enrolment rate
R10.	Patient members → Revenues from industry → Patient organization's revenues → Patient organization's cumulated earnings → Paid volunteers → Volunteers in outpatient clinic → Patient organization's administrative service → Effect of outpatient service quality improvement on enrolment rate → Enrolment rate

increment of patient organization's revenues and cumulated earnings, creating financial resources eventually allocable to hire new 'paid volunteers'. B1 shows the effect of new 'paid volunteers' on 'patient organization costs', thereby reducing cumulated earnings. B2 illustrates the effect of paid volunteers allocated to merchandising campaigns on patient organization's costs. More 'paid volunteers' will allow more 'volunteers in merchandising' and the purchasing of more 'merchandising gadgets', which will have a depletive effect on 'patient organization's earnings'.

The SFD of the sector of 'Patient co-created healthcare' (figure 12) highlights nine interacting loops. All of them are reinforcing and numbered from R12 to R20 (see table 4). Loop R12 integrates perceived quality, trust

Table 3. Patient organization's financial performances: causal loops

LOOP	LOOP VARIABLES
R11.	Paid volunteers → Volunteers in merchandising → Merchandising gadgets → Revenues from merchandising → Patient organization's revenues → Patient organization's cumulated earnings
B1.	Paid volunteers → Patient organization' costs → Patient organization's cumulated earnings
B2.	Paid volunteers → Volunteers in merchandising → Merchandising gadgets → Costs of merchandising → Patient organization's cumulated earnings

and adherence to recommended treatments. A positive 'change in perceived quality of healthcare' causes an increase of 'trust in healthcare', which in turn boosts the 'adherence skills to recommended treatments', thereby decreasing the 'gap in patient adherence skills'. The less is such gap the more will be the 'fulfilled therapy requirements', able to feedback to a further improvement to the perceived quality of healthcare.

Loop 13 shows how 'healthcare literacy' and 'patient knowledge on own symptoms' mutually reinforce each other. R14 refers to the physicians' learning from experience: the 'clinical knowledge about disease' gained through facing specific cohorts of medical cases, progressively result in a wider 'cumulated clinical experience'. In turn it will increase the 'clinical knowledge about disease' by helping to solve new clinical cases.

Loop R15 portrays patients' knowledge and reported knowledge self-reinforcing dynamics. More and better quality of 'patient reported information

Figure 12. Causal loop diagram regarding patient co-created healthcare

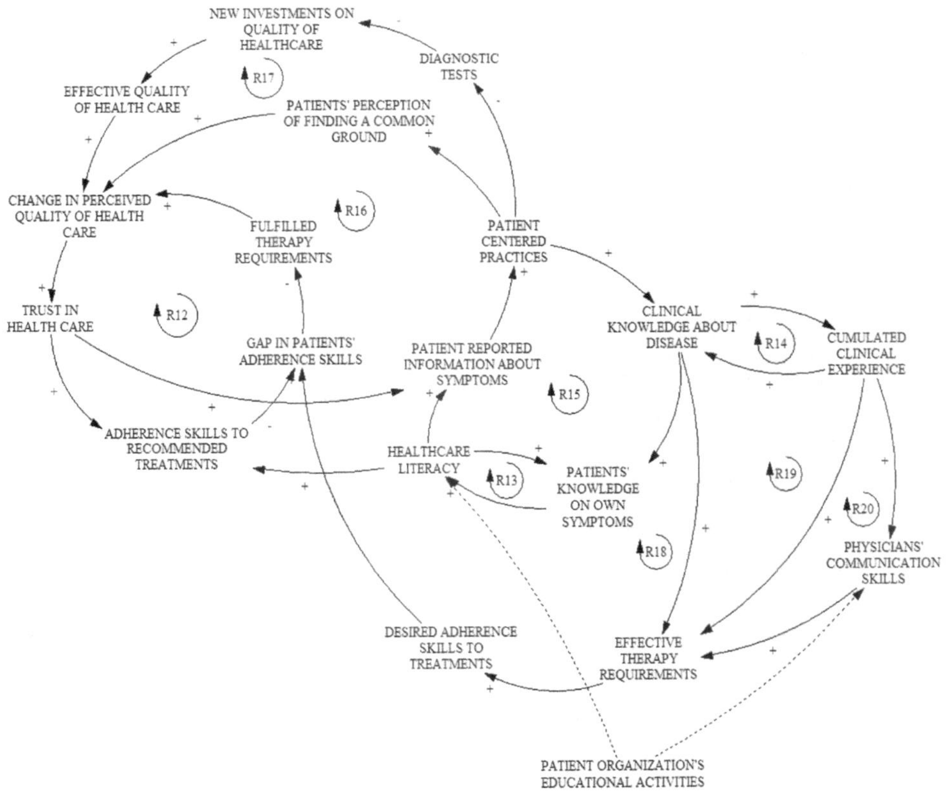

about symptoms' will result in a rise of 'patient-centered practices', which in turn will increase the 'clinical knowledge about disease'. The information will be transferred to patients, that will enlarge their 'knowledge on own symptoms' and their 'healthcare literacy', consenting them to increase the 'patient reported information about symptoms'.

Loop 16 depicts that 'trust in healthcare' affects 'patient reported information about symptoms' and, again 'patient-centered practices'. This fact causes the rise of 'patient perception of finding a common ground', which feeds back into 'trust in healthcare'.

In line with researches about positive financial impacts of patient-centered practices (Charmel & Frampton, 2008), R17 depicts the chain effect of trust on perceived quality through patient-centered practices and diagnostic test reduction. An increase of 'trust in healthcare' contributes positively to 'patient reported information about symptoms' and then 'patient centered-practices'. The latter deters the variable 'diagnostic tests', which elapses savings for 'new investments on quality of healthcare', provoking 'change in perceived quality of healthcare' and re-stimulating trust. Loops R18 and R19 present a

Table 4. Sector of Patient co-created Healthcare: causal loops

LOOP	VARIABLES
R12.	Change in perceived quality of healthcare → Trust in healthcare → Adherence skills to recommended treatments → Gap in patients' adherence skills → Fulfilled therapy requirements
R13.	Healthcare literacy → Patients' knowledge on own symptom
R14.	Clinical knowledge about disease → Cumulated clinical experience
R15.	Patient reported information about symptoms → Patient centered practices → Clinical knowledge about disease → Patients' knowledge on own symptoms → Healthcare literacy
R16.	Trust in healthcare → Patient reported information about symptoms → Patient centered practices → Patients' perception of finding a common ground
R17.	Trust in healthcare → Patient reported information about symptoms → Patient centered practices → Diagnostic tests → New investments on quality of healthcare → Change in perceived quality of healthcare
R18.	Trust in healthcare → Patient reported information about symptoms → Patient centered practices → Clinical knowledge about disease → Effective therapy requirements → Desired adherence skills to treatments → Gap in patients' adherence skills →Fulfilled therapy requirements → Change in perceived quality of healthcare
R19.	Trust in healthcare → Patient reported information about symptoms → Patient centered practices → Clinical knowledge about disease → Cumulated clinical experience → Effective therapy requirements → Desired adherence skills to treatments → Gap in patients' adherence skills →Fulfilled therapy requirements → Change in perceived quality of healthcare
R20.	Trust in healthcare → Patient reported information about symptoms → Patient centered practices → Clinical knowledge about disease → Cumulated clinical experience → Physicians' communication skills → Effective therapy requirements → Desired adherence skills to treatments → Gap in patients' adherence skills →Fulfilled therapy requirements → Change in perceived quality of healthcare

chain effect of trust on perceived quality through, among the others, patient-centered practices and effective therapy requirements.

In R18, a trigger of 'trust in healthcare' stimulates 'patient reported information about symptoms' and 'patient-centered practices'. The latter variable increases the 'clinical knowledge about disease', that contribute to 'effective therapy requirements'. From them, there derive certain 'desired adherence skills to treatments', which, compared to the stock of actual skills, result in a lower 'gap in patient adherence skills'. This means an increase of the stock of 'fulfilled therapy requirements' and in a 'change in perceived quality of healthcare'.

R19 presents similar dynamics, except for the inclusion of the 'cumulated clinical experience' within the circuit. Finally, loop R20, integrates the effect of 'cumulated clinical experience' (together with educational paths), 'physicians' communication skills' and 'effective therapy requirements'.

Simulations

The model was built using a simulation software (iThink by Stella), suitable for the building of the stock-and-flow structure, paired with a set of differential equations representative of decision rules and behavioral relationships. So far, this activity of quantitative formalization concerned the sectors 'delivery of healthcare' and 'patient organization's management'. On the contrary, the 'patient co-created healthcare' sector still lays at a qualitative modelling stage, since it requires supplementary work for parameter estimation and tests.

However, the model built up to now allows to simulate relevant variables' patterns over the time, in response to alternative policies. The simulations were performed within a 10-year timeframe (from time 1 to 11), and according to six policy scenarios (summarized in table 5), characterized by different allocations of volunteers in outpatient clinic and in merchandising activities.

In scenario 1 (baseline), the patient organization has 9 paid volunteers, 4 of them working in outpatient clinic and 5 employed in merchandising. In the second and third scenarios, an outpatient policy is activated with different intensities (by doubling and tripling the volunteers in the outpatient clinic) keeping constant the volunteers in merchandising. The scenario 4 imagines a merchandising policy, by adding three units to the volunteers to merchandise. Finally, scenarios 5 and 6 presents two possible mix of outpatient and merchandising policies.

In the baseline scenario (figure 13) the stock variable 'waiting list', after a slightly declining behaviour, is characterized by a steady growth. This is because, excepting for the period from time 1 to time 3, its outflow 'to outpatient clinic' is always below the inflow, revealing capacity constraints in the system.

Simulations have been carried on by monitoring key-variables:

- In the sector 'delivery of healthcare': the simulated variables were the stocks 'waiting list' and 'outpatients', as well as their difference, indicated by the auxiliary variable 'unsatisfied demand';
- In the sector 'patient organization's management' the simulations regarded the stock 'cumulated patient members' and its inflow 'enrolment rate'.

The simulated policies in figure 14 shows that the outpatient policy has a relevant effect reducing waiting list, increasing outpatients and thus lowering the unsatisfied demand. On the other side, the merchandising policy alone (line 4), or in combination with the outpatient policy (lines 5 and 6) is basically ineffective on the sector of healthcare delivery. This result does not surprise, since none of the loops regarding the administrative tasks performed by volunteers in outpatient clinic (R2-R10) involve an effect of merchandising campaigns on outpatient capacity. This does not necessarily mean that the merchandising activity is useless for patient organizations and for healthcare provision. Looking at the sector of 'patient organization's management', the simulated behaviours in figure 15 show that each of the suggested policy can trigger the 'enrolment rate' and by this way the 'cumulated patient members'. However, the merchandising policy alone (line 4), even producing

Table 5. Alternative policy scenarios

SIMULATED POLICY SCENARIOS	A) VOLUNTEERS IN OUTPATIENT CLINIC	B) VOLUNTEERS TO MERCHANDISE	NUMBER OF VOLUNTEERS (A+B)
1	4	5	9
2	8	5	13
3	12	5	**17**
4	4	8	12
5	12	8	**20**
6	8	9	**17**

Figure 13. Baseline simulation of waiting list and related flows

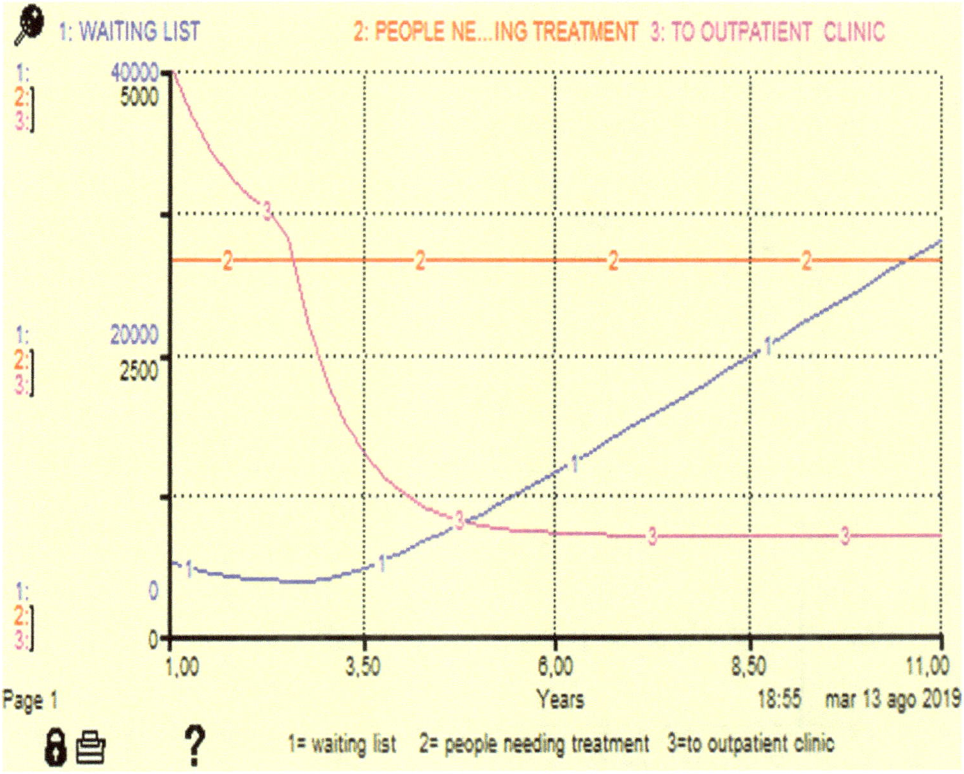

an enlargement of membership, is the less effective. The outpatient policies (lines 2 and 3) presents better enrolment and membership performances than mixed policies.

The mixed policies (lines 5 and 6) provoke a dramatic performance difference in comparison to the other options, as it is also possible to account in figure 16. Policy 6 produces the greatest values in terms of enrolment rate and cumulated members and is also the most efficient policy. Indeed, with 3 paid volunteers less than policy 5, it can produce an enrolment rate's performance gap of more than the 20% in the first three years, after then diminishing over the time up the 3%. Re-looking at table 5, it is worth noticing the same number of paid volunteers in policy 6 and 3, but their simulated outputs are sensibly different, with percentual gaps overcoming the 100%. This means that patient organizations need to properly plan an efficient use of human resources, not neglecting any of their strategic areas. Policy 6 has

Figure 14. Delivery of healthcare: scenario analysis

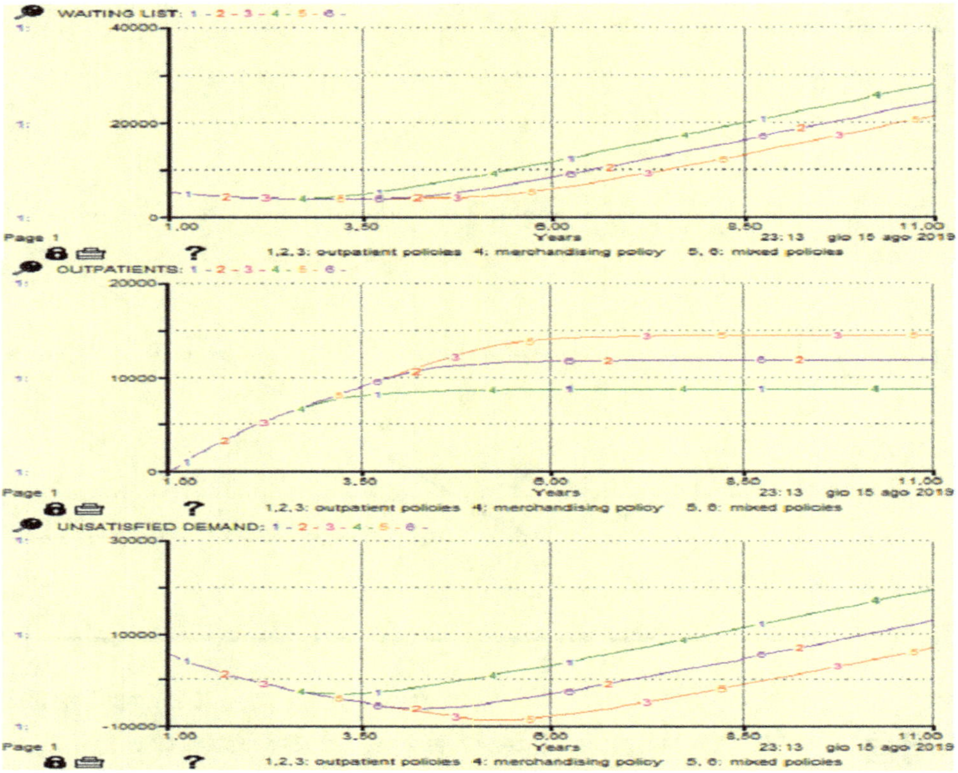

also the merit to make all the loops regarding the development dynamics of the patient organization (i.e. the ones in table 2) working favourably.

By simulating behaviours occurring in different 'places' of the system, it is possible to shed light into the effects of alternative policies, avoiding unintended consequences and allowing a better use of financial and human resources. In addition, it can be envisaged a trade-off between public and private interests and policy preferences. Indeed, the third scenario, with 12 volunteers employed in outpatient clinic, produces the best results in terms of healthcare provision, and then it would be the most suitable policy from the perspective of public healthcare provider. On the other hand, in patient organization's view, the best suited policy would be the sixth, in consideration that membership is a relevant component of its budget, allowing to cover expenses, included compensations for volunteers. In order to align such conflicting interests, it could be suggested (if consented by regulations), a corrective financial intervention from public decision makers, for example

Figure 15. Patient organization's management: scenario analysis

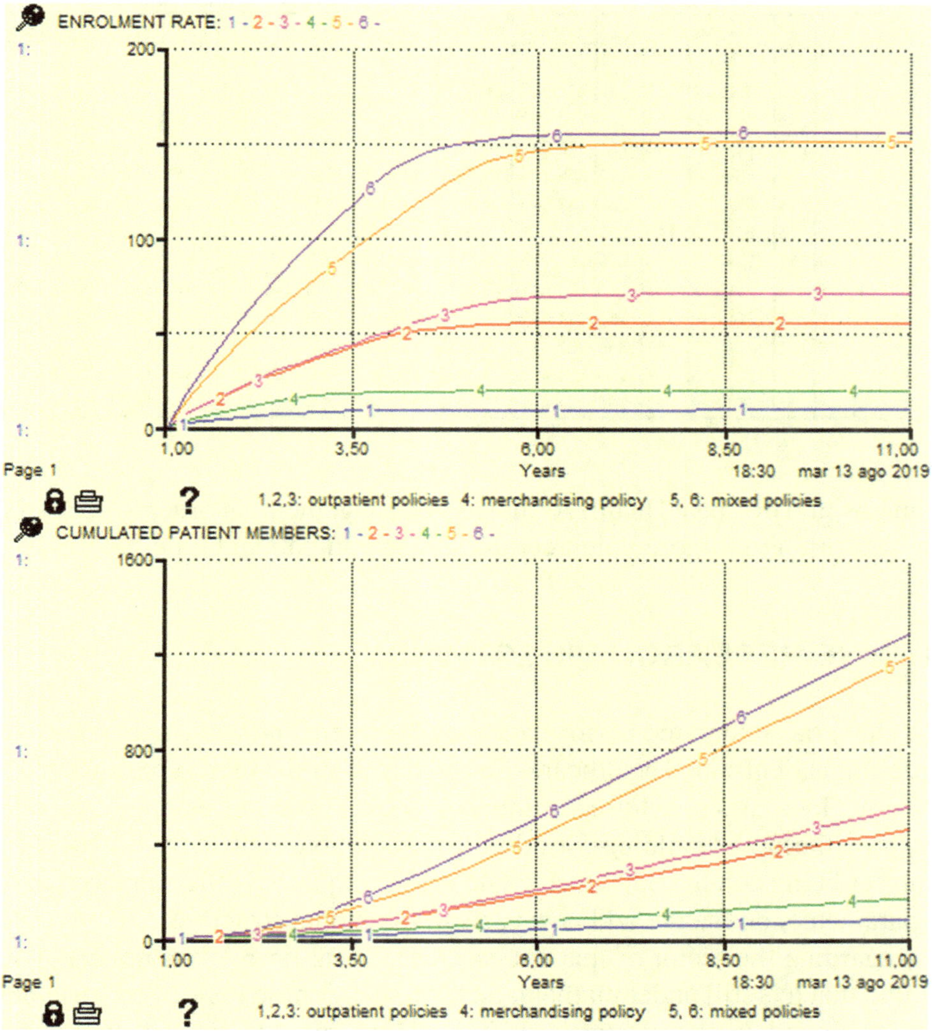

Figure 16. Enroment rate and cumulated patient members' simulated outputs

	ENROLMENT RATE								CUMULATED PATIENT MEMBERS							
scenarios	1	2	3	4	5	6	gap 3-6	gap 5-6	1	2	3	4	5	6	gap 3-6	gap 5-6
time																
0	2	8	9	4	18	23	171,73%	26,69%	2	8	9	4	18	23	171,73%	26,69%
1	6	26	27	12	58	74	171,59%	26,66%	7	34	36	16	77	97	171,59%	26,65%
2	8	40	42	17	90	114	171,63%	26,66%	15	75	78	33	166	211	171,65%	26,66%
3	9	51	55	18	118	142	158,21%	20,41%	24	125	133	51	285	353	166,06%	24,06%
4	9	54	65	19	140	152	132,54%	8,43%	32	179	198	70	425	505	154,99%	18,90%
5	9	55	69	19	148	155	124,34%	4,61%	41	234	267	88	573	660	147,07%	15,21%
6	9	55	70	19	150	156	122,20%	3,61%	50	289	337	107	723	816	141,90%	12,80%
7	9	55	70	19	151	156	121,64%	3,35%	59	345	408	126	874	972	138,41%	11,17%
8	9	55	70	19	151	156	121,48%	3,27%	67	400	478	145	1025	1128	135,91%	10,00%
9	9	55	70	19	151	156	121,43%	3,25%	76	455	548	163	1176	1284	134,05%	9,14%
10	9	55	70	19	151	156	121,41%	3,25%	85	511	619	182	1327	1440	132,61%	8,47%
11	9	55	70	19	151	156	121,41%	3,24%	94	566	689	201	1478	1596	131,47%	7,93%

from hospital or Local Health Authority's management, in order to cover the compensation of 4 more volunteer units in the outpatient clinic.

FUTURE RESEARCH DIRECTIONS

The study has integrated performance management and system dynamics to represent patient-aided healthcare. The resulting model represents a complex dynamic hypothesis, whose testing is ongoing. Next research steps will complete the model building considering the outputs of statistic and sensitivity analyses being conducted, which could lead to adjust existing equations and/or parameters or even to add new parts to the model structure.

Regarding the sector of 'patient co-created healthcare', it is important to remind that it is still under mathematic formalization, so none of its variables were included in the scenario analysis. However, the related qualitative diagrams were inserted in the chapter, considering them useful to gain deep insights. Future researches could enlarge model boundaries by deepening the financial aspects (in particular, the budgeting processes), for both healthcare providers and patient organizations. Further modelling efforts may also involve the assignments of public and industrial funds to healthcare organizations, depicting trade-offs and potential conflicts of interests. Finally, new studies could deal with patient contributions to other health-related aspects, such as research and development and healthcare policy making.

CONCLUSION

The chapter has shown how to build a dynamic performance management system able to capture relevant management dynamics occurring within patient organizations and patient-aided health provision. The modelling has been conducted by integrating qualitative (SFD and CLD) and quantitative (computer simulations) tools. The first ones had the merit to show systemic mechanisms of accumulation and feedback. The simulations allowed what-if analyses in pace with different allocative scenarios of human resources. Such methodological approach can help in re-thinking the totality of the patient-aided healthcare, providing private and public decision-makers (also belonging to different organizations), to gain a shared understanding of public service provisions. Looking at the entire system and capturing the links between its parts, the model (together with its future developments) could detect policies' unintended consequences, and force policy makers to find collaborative solutions to public issues, thus promoting effective networked governances.

REFERENCES

Altin, S. V., & Stock, S. (2015). Impact of health literacy, accessibility and coordination of care on patient's satisfaction with primary care in Germany. *BMC Family Practice*, *16*(1), 148–154. doi:10.118612875-015-0372-0 PMID:26492959

Barry, M. J., & Edgman-Levitan, S. (2012). Shared Decision Making The Pinnacle of Patient-Centered Care. *The New England Journal of Medicine*, *366*(9), 780–781. doi:10.1056/NEJMp1109283 PMID:22375967

Berghout, M., Van Exel, J., Leensvaart, L., & Cramm, J. M. (2015). Healthcare professionals' views on patient-centered care in hospitals. *BMC Health Services Research*, *15*(1), 385–397. doi:10.118612913-015-1049-z PMID:26373841

Bertakis, K. D., & Azari, R. (2011). Patient-Centered Care is Associated with Decreased Healthcare Utilization. *Journal of the American Board of Family Medicine*, *24*(3), 229–239. doi:10.3122/jabfm.2011.03.100170 PMID:21551394

Bianchi, C. (2010). Improving performance and fostering accountability in the Public Sector through System Dynamics modelling. From 'external' to an 'internal' perspective. *Systems Research and Behavioral Science*, *27*(4), 361–384. doi:10.1002res.1038

Bianchi, C. (2012). Enhancing Performance Management and Sustainable Organizational Growth through System Dynamics Modeling. In S. N. Groesser & R. Zeier (Eds.), *Systemic Management for Intelligent Organizations: Concepts, Model-Based Approaches, and Applications* (pp. 143–161). Heidelberg, Germany: Springer. doi:10.1007/978-3-642-29244-6_8

Charmel, P. A., & Frampton, S. B. (2008, Mar.). Building the business case for patient-centered care. *Healthcare Financial Management*, 1–8. PMID:19097611

Davis, K., Schoenbaum, S. C., & Audet, A. M. (2005). A 2020 Vision of Patient-Centered Primary Care. *Journal of General Internal Medicine*, *20*(10), 953–954. doi:10.1111/j.1525-1497.2005.0178.x PMID:16191145

Elg, M., Engstrom, J., Witell, L., & Poksinska, B. (2012). Co-creation and learning in health-care service development. *Journal of Service Management*, *23*(3), 328–343. doi:10.1108/09564231211248435

Epstein, R. M., & Street, R. L. (2011). The Values and Value of Patient-Centered Care. *Annals of Family Medicine*, *9*(2), 100–103. doi:10.1370/afm.1239 PMID:21403134

Fiorio, C. V., Gorli, M., & Verzillo, S. (2018). Evaluating organizational change in healthcare: The patient-centered hospital model. *BMC Health Services Research*, *18*(1), 95–109. doi:10.118612913-018-2877-4 PMID:29422045

Fiscella, K., Meldrum, S., Franks, P., Shields, C. G., Duberstein, P., McDaniel, S., & Epstein, R. M. (2004). Patient Trust. Is It Related to Patient-Centered Behavior of Primary Care Physicians? *Medical Care*, *42*(11), 1049–1055. doi:10.1097/00005650-200411000-00003 PMID:15586831

Ford-Gilboe, M., Wathen, C. N., Varcoe, C., Herbert, C., Jackson, B. E., Lavoie, C. J., ... Browne, A. J. (2018). How Equity-Oriented Healthcare Affects Health: Key Mechanisms and Implications for Primary Healthcare Practice and Policy. *The Milbank Quarterly*, 635–671. doi:10.1111/1468-0009.12349 PMID:30350420

Forrester, J. W. (1961). *Industrial Dynamics*. Boston, MA: The MIT Press.

Hoffman, T. C., Montori, V. M., & Del Mar, C. (2014). The Connection Between Evidence-Based Medicine and Shared Decision Making. *Journal of the American Medical Association, 312*(13), 1295–1296. doi:10.1001/jama.2014.10186 PMID:25268434

Inamdar, N., Kaplan, R.S., & Bower, M. (2002). Applying the balanced scorecard in healthcare provider organizations. *Journal of Healthcare Management/American College of Healthcare Executives, 47*(3), 179-196.

Kane, P. M., Murtagh, F. E. M., Ryan, K., Mahon, N. G., McAdam, B., McQuillan, R., ... Daveson, B. A. (2015). The gap between policy and practice: A systematic review of patient-centred care interventions in chronic heart failure. *Health Fail Review, 20*(6), 673–687. doi:10.100710741-015-9508-5 PMID:26435042

Kaplan, R. S., & Norton, D. P. (1992). The balance scorecard: Measures that drive performance. *Harvard Business Review, 70*(1-2), 71–79. PMID:10119714

Kim, C., Wright, F. C., Look Hong, N. J., Groot, G., Helyer, L., Meiers, P., ... Gagliardi, A. R. (2017). Patient and provider experiences with active surveillance: A scoping review. *PLoS One, 13*(2), 1–17. PMID:29401514

Luxford, K., Safran, D. G., & Delbanco, T. (2011). Promoting patient-centered care: A qualitative study of facilitators and barriers in healthcare organizations with a reputation for improving the patient experience. *International Journal for Quality in Health Care, 23*(5), 510–515. doi:10.1093/intqhc/mzr024 PMID:21586433

Mc Lean, K. A., Drake, T. M., Sgrò, A., Camilleri-Brennan, J., Knight, S. R., Ots, R., ... Harrison, E. M. (2019). The effect of liver transplantation on patient-centred outcomes: A propensity-scorematched analysis. *Transplant International, 32*(8), 808–819. PMID:30793373

McCabe, R., & Healey, P. G. T. (2018). Miscommunication in Doctor–Patient Communication. *Topics in Cognitive Science, 10*(2), 409–424. doi:10.1111/tops.12337 PMID:29749042

McCaffrey, S. A., Chiauzzi, E., Chan, C., & Hoole, M. (2018). Understanding 'Good Healthcare' from the Patient's Perspective: Development of a Conceptual Model Using Group Concept Mapping. *The Patient-Centered Outcomes Research, 12*(1), 83–95. doi:10.100740271-018-0320-x

Prag, P., Wittek, R., & Mills, M. C. (2017). The educational gradient in self-rated health in Europe: Does the doctor–patient relationship make a difference? *Acta Sociologica*, *60*(4), 325–341. doi:10.1177/0001699316670715

Rathert, C., Wyrwich, M. D., & Boren, S. A. (2013). Patient-centered care and outcomes a systematic review of the literature. *Medical Care Research and Review: MCRR*, *70*(4), 351–379. doi:10.1177/1077558712465774 PMID:23169897

Richardson, G. P. (2011). Reflections on the foundations of system dynamics. *System Dynamics Review*, *27*(3), 219–243. doi:10.1002dr.462

Santana, M. J., Manalili, K., Jolley, R. J., Zelinsky, S., Quan, H., & Lu, M. (2017). How to practice person-centred care: A conceptual framework. *Health Expectations*, *21*(2), 429–440. doi:10.1111/hex.12640 PMID:29151269

Sarango, M., Hohl, C., Gonzalez, N., Palmeros, A., Powell, M. L., & Hirsch, M. (2018). Strategies to Build a Patient-Centered Medical Home for Multiply Diagnosed People Living With HIV Who Are Experiencing Homelessness or Unstable Housing. *American Journal of Public Health*, *108*(7), 519–521. doi:10.2105/AJPH.2018.304675

Scholl, I., Zill, J. M., Harter, M., & Dirmaier, J. (2014). An integrative model of patient centeredness? A systematic review and concept analysis. *PLoS One*, *9*(9), 1–9. doi:10.1371/journal.pone.0107828 PMID:25229640

Selby, J. V., & Lipstein, S. H. (2014). PCORI at 3 years. Progress, lessons, and plans. *The New England Journal of Medicine*, *370*(7), 592–595. doi:10.1056/NEJMp1313061 PMID:24521104

Sepucha, K.R., Fowler, F.J. Jr., & Mulley, A.G Jr. (2004). Policy Support For Patient-Centered Care: The Need For Measurable Improvements In Decision Quality. *Health Affairs*, 54-62.

Shippee, N. D., Shah, N. D., May, C. L., Mair, F. S., & Montori, V. M. (2012). Cumulative complexity: A functional, patient-centered model of patient complexity can improve research and practice. *Journal of Clinical Epidemiology*, *65*(10), 1041–1051. doi:10.1016/j.jclinepi.2012.05.005 PMID:22910536

Sterman, J. D. (2000). *Business Dynamics. System thinking and modeling for a complex world.* Boston, MA: Mc Graw-Hill.

Stewart, M., Brown, J. B., Donner, A., McWhinney, I. R., Oates, J., & Weston, W. (2000). The Impact of Patient-Centered Care on Outcomes. *The Journal of Family Practice*, *49*(9), 796–804. PMID:11032203

Terry, G., & Kayes, N. (2019). Person centered care in neurorehabilitation: A secondary analysis. *Disability and Rehabilitation*, 1–10. doi:10.1080/09638288.2018.1561952 PMID:30696295

Verwijmeren, D., & Grootens, K. (2018). Shared decision making in pharmacotherapy decisions, perceived by patients with bipolar disorder. *International Journal of Bipolar Disorders*, *6*(1), 21–28. doi:10.118640345-018-0129-5 PMID:30284089

KEY TERMS AND DEFINITIONS

Dynamic Performance Management Framework: Model building framework combining performance management and system dynamics.

System Dynamics: Simulation methodology suitable to deal with dynamic problems (i.e., issue behaviors occurring over the time) in complex social, economic, or ecological systems.

Related Readings

To continue IGI Global's long-standing tradition of advancing innovation through emerging research, please find below a compiled list of recommended IGI Global book chapters and journal articles in the areas of healthcare systems, patient care, and public healthcare. These related readings will provide additional information and guidance to further enrich your knowledge and assist you with your own research.

Allison, K., & Allison, C. (2017). Mental Illness, Youth, and Lessons from Residential Treatment Centers. In V. Bryan & J. Bird (Eds.), *Healthcare Community Synergism between Patients, Practitioners, and Researchers* (pp. 126–151). Hershey, PA: IGI Global. doi:10.4018/978-1-5225-0640-9.ch007

Alsalamah, S., Alsalamah, H., Gray, A. W., & Hilton, J. (2016). Information Security Threats in Patient-Centred Healthcare. In A. Moumtzoglou (Ed.), *M-Health Innovations for Patient-Centered Care* (pp. 298–318). Hershey, PA: IGI Global. doi:10.4018/978-1-4666-9861-1.ch015

Altinpulluk, H., & Kurubacak, G. (2016). MoBip Project: To Raise Awareness about Bipolar Disorder through an 3D Pop-Up Book. In A. Moumtzoglou (Ed.), *M-Health Innovations for Patient-Centered Care* (pp. 147–169). Hershey, PA: IGI Global. doi:10.4018/978-1-4666-9861-1.ch008

Anastasiou, A., Giokas, K., Koutsouri, G., & Iliopoulou, D. (2017). Intelligent Medication Adherence Monitoring System. In A. Moumtzoglou (Ed.), *Design, Development, and Integration of Reliable Electronic Healthcare Platforms* (pp. 72–85). Hershey, PA: IGI Global. doi:10.4018/978-1-5225-1724-5.ch004

Arling, P. A., Miech, E. J., & Arling, G. W. (2017). Improving Quality Improvement Collaboratives: Mixing Communication Media to Attain Multiple Measures of Success. In A. Moumtzoglou (Ed.), *Design, Development, and Integration of Reliable Electronic Healthcare Platforms* (pp. 243–254). Hershey, PA: IGI Global. doi:10.4018/978-1-5225-1724-5.ch014

Arnan, P., & Adugu, E. (2016). Individual, Institutional, and Environmental Factors Promoting Patient Retention and Dropout. In G. Graffigna (Ed.), *Promoting Patient Engagement and Participation for Effective Healthcare Reform* (pp. 41–57). Hershey, PA: IGI Global. doi:10.4018/978-1-4666-9992-2.ch003

Becker, L. C. (2016). Habilitation, Healthy Agency, and Patient-Participation. In G. Graffigna (Ed.), *Promoting Patient Engagement and Participation for Effective Healthcare Reform* (pp. 1–24). Hershey, PA: IGI Global. doi:10.4018/978-1-4666-9992-2.ch001

Bello-Bravo, J., Lutomia, A. N., Songu, T., & Pittendrigh, B. R. (2017). Viral Education via Mobile Phone: Virtual International Networks and Ebola Prevention in Sierra Leone. In K. Moahi, K. Bwalya, & P. Sebina (Eds.), *Health Information Systems and the Advancement of Medical Practice in Developing Countries* (pp. 78–92). Hershey, PA: IGI Global. doi:10.4018/978-1-5225-2262-1.ch005

Binhadyan, B., & Wickramasinghe, N. (2016). An Investigation of the Role of Using IS/IT in the Delivery of Treatments for ADHD in University Students. In T. Iyamu & A. Tatnall (Eds.), *Maximizing Healthcare Delivery and Management through Technology Integration* (pp. 58–75). Hershey, PA: IGI Global. doi:10.4018/978-1-4666-9446-0.ch005

Bird, J. L. (2017). Writing Healing Narratives. In V. Bryan & J. Bird (Eds.), *Healthcare Community Synergism between Patients, Practitioners, and Researchers* (pp. 1–28). Hershey, PA: IGI Global. doi:10.4018/978-1-5225-0640-9.ch001

Bougoulias, K., Kouris, I., Prasinos, M., Giokas, K., & Koutsouris, D. (2017). Ob/Gyn EMR Software: A Solution for Obstetricians and Gynecologists. In A. Moumtzoglou (Ed.), *Design, Development, and Integration of Reliable Electronic Healthcare Platforms* (pp. 101–111). Hershey, PA: IGI Global. doi:10.4018/978-1-5225-1724-5.ch006

Bourek, A. (2017). How to Make Your Work Really Influence Future Healthcare: From Projects through Policies to Integration into Health Systems. In A. Moumtzoglou (Ed.), *Design, Development, and Integration of Reliable Electronic Healthcare Platforms* (pp. 271–296). Hershey, PA: IGI Global. doi:10.4018/978-1-5225-1724-5.ch016

Bruscaglioni, L. (2016). No Entry: Prohibitions and Violations in Organizational Spaces across the Patient-Staff Interface in Hospital. In G. Graffigna (Ed.), *Promoting Patient Engagement and Participation for Effective Healthcare Reform* (pp. 171–191). Hershey, PA: IGI Global. doi:10.4018/978-1-4666-9992-2.ch009

Bwalya, K. J. (2017). Next Wave of Tele-Medicine: Virtual Presence of Medical Personnel. In K. Moahi, K. Bwalya, & P. Sebina (Eds.), *Health Information Systems and the Advancement of Medical Practice in Developing Countries* (pp. 168–180). Hershey, PA: IGI Global. doi:10.4018/978-1-5225-2262-1.ch010

Calogero, A., Longo, F., Nicoletti, L., & Padovano, A. (2017). Evaluating the Impacts of Lean Management Practices in Healthcare via Simulation. *International Journal of Privacy and Health Information Management*, *5*(1), 1–22. doi:10.4018/IJPHIM.2017010101

Chakraborty, C., Gupta, B., & Ghosh, S. K. (2016). Mobile Telemedicine Systems for Remote Patient's Chronic Wound Monitoring. In A. Moumtzoglou (Ed.), *M-Health Innovations for Patient-Centered Care* (pp. 213–239). Hershey, PA: IGI Global. doi:10.4018/978-1-4666-9861-1.ch011

Chavez, A., & Kovarik, C. (2017). Open Source Technology for Medical Practice in Developing Countries. In K. Moahi, K. Bwalya, & P. Sebina (Eds.), *Health Information Systems and the Advancement of Medical Practice in Developing Countries* (pp. 33–59). Hershey, PA: IGI Global. doi:10.4018/978-1-5225-2262-1.ch003

Costarides, V., Zygomalas, A., Giokas, K., & Koutsouris, D. (2017). Robotics in Surgical Techniques: Present and Future Trends. In A. Moumtzoglou (Ed.), *Design, Development, and Integration of Reliable Electronic Healthcare Platforms* (pp. 86–100). Hershey, PA: IGI Global. doi:10.4018/978-1-5225-1724-5.ch005

Czarnecka, K. H., & Pawliczak, F. (2018). Managed Healthcare: A Temporary Trend or a New Standard for Providing Health Services? In A. Rosiek-Kryszewska & K. Leksowski (Eds.), *Healthcare Administration for Patient Safety and Engagement* (pp. 1–12). Hershey, PA: IGI Global. doi:10.4018/978-1-5225-3946-9.ch001

Darcy, N., Perera, S., Stanley, G., Rumisha, S., Assenga, K., Polycarp, F., ... Teesdale, S. (2017). Case Study: The Tanzania Health Facility Registry. In K. Moahi, K. Bwalya, & P. Sebina (Eds.), *Health Information Systems and the Advancement of Medical Practice in Developing Countries* (pp. 208–236). Hershey, PA: IGI Global. doi:10.4018/978-1-5225-2262-1.ch013

Donato, S., & Bertoni, A. (2016). A Relational Perspective on Patient Engagement: Suggestions from Couple-Based Research and Intervention. In G. Graffigna (Ed.), *Promoting Patient Engagement and Participation for Effective Healthcare Reform* (pp. 83–106). Hershey, PA: IGI Global. doi:10.4018/978-1-4666-9992-2.ch005

Dotson, E., Hibbler, D. K., & Scott, L. (2017). Culture of Learning Cities: Connecting Leisure and Health for Lifelong Learning Communities. In V. Bryan & J. Bird (Eds.), *Healthcare Community Synergism between Patients, Practitioners, and Researchers* (pp. 152–175). Hershey, PA: IGI Global. doi:10.4018/978-1-5225-0640-9.ch008

Drowos, J. L., & Wood, S. K. (2017). Preparing Future Physicians to Adapt to the Changing Health Care System: Promoting Humanism through Curricular Design. In V. Bryan & J. Bird (Eds.), *Healthcare Community Synergism between Patients, Practitioners, and Researchers* (pp. 106–125). Hershey, PA: IGI Global. doi:10.4018/978-1-5225-0640-9.ch006

Edoh, T. O., Pawar, P. A., Brügge, B., & Teege, G. (2016). A Multidisciplinary Remote Healthcare Delivery System to Increase Health Care Access, Pathology Screening, and Treatment in Developing Countries: The Case of Benin. *International Journal of Healthcare Information Systems and Informatics, 11*(4), 1–31. doi:10.4018/IJHISI.2016100101

Ellington, L., & Bryan, V. C. (2017). Incognito: The Neuroscience of Grief and Grieving. In V. Bryan & J. Bird (Eds.), *Healthcare Community Synergism between Patients, Practitioners, and Researchers* (pp. 272–291). Hershey, PA: IGI Global. doi:10.4018/978-1-5225-0640-9.ch012

Estrella, P., & Tsourakis, N. (2017). Migrating from ISO/IEC 9126 to SQUARE: A Case Study on the Evaluation of Medical Speech Translation Systems. In A. Moumtzoglou (Ed.), *Design, Development, and Integration of Reliable Electronic Healthcare Platforms* (pp. 160–178). Hershey, PA: IGI Global. doi:10.4018/978-1-5225-1724-5.ch010

Faruq, Q. O. (2016). General Practitioners' Adoption and Use of ICT. In T. Iyamu & A. Tatnall (Eds.), *Maximizing Healthcare Delivery and Management through Technology Integration* (pp. 152–168). Hershey, PA: IGI Global. doi:10.4018/978-1-4666-9446-0.ch010

Gaspar, R., Domingos, S., Diniz, A. M., & Falanga, R. (2016). Barriers to and Facilitators of Older Adult's Adherence to Health Recommendations: Towards an Engaging Two-way Health Communication. In G. Graffigna (Ed.), *Promoting Patient Engagement and Participation for Effective Healthcare Reform* (pp. 58–82). Hershey, PA: IGI Global. doi:10.4018/978-1-4666-9992-2.ch004

Giokas, K., Costarides, V., & Koutsouris, D. (2016). Integrated Platform for the Lifestyle Change and Holistic Approach to Personalized Prevention and Self-Management of Patients with High Blood Pressure. In A. Moumtzoglou (Ed.), *M-Health Innovations for Patient-Centered Care* (pp. 72–90). Hershey, PA: IGI Global. doi:10.4018/978-1-4666-9861-1.ch004

Giokas, K., Katrakazas, P., & Koutsouris, D. (2016). A Collaborative m-Health Platform for Evidence-Based Self-Management and Detection of Chronic Multimorbidity Development and Progression. In A. Moumtzoglou (Ed.), *M-Health Innovations for Patient-Centered Care* (pp. 52–71). Hershey, PA: IGI Global. doi:10.4018/978-1-4666-9861-1.ch003

Gorli, M., Liberati, E. G., Galuppo, L., & Scaratti, G. (2016). The Patient Centered Organizational Model in Italian Hospitals: Practical Challenges for Patient Engagement. In G. Graffigna (Ed.), *Promoting Patient Engagement and Participation for Effective Healthcare Reform* (pp. 152–170). Hershey, PA: IGI Global. doi:10.4018/978-1-4666-9992-2.ch008

Graffigna, G., & Barello, S. (2016). The Value of Measuring Patient Engagement in Healthcare: New Frontiers for Healthcare Quality. In G. Graffigna (Ed.), *Promoting Patient Engagement and Participation for Effective Healthcare Reform* (pp. 192–214). Hershey, PA: IGI Global. doi:10.4018/978-1-4666-9992-2.ch010

Hamunyela, S., & Iyamu, T. (2016). Healthcare Services for Nomadics through a Mobile Framework. In T. Iyamu & A. Tatnall (Eds.), *Maximizing Healthcare Delivery and Management through Technology Integration* (pp. 46–57). Hershey, PA: IGI Global. doi:10.4018/978-1-4666-9446-0.ch004

Han-Lin, C., Yang, A. W., Pittayachawan, S., & Wickramasinghe, N. (2016). An Analysis on the Utilisation of Health Information Technology to Support Clinical Operation of Chinese Medicine. In T. Iyamu & A. Tatnall (Eds.), *Maximizing Healthcare Delivery and Management through Technology Integration* (pp. 113–132). Hershey, PA: IGI Global. doi:10.4018/978-1-4666-9446-0.ch008

Handayani, P. W., Sandhyaduhita, P. I., Hidayanto, A. N., Pinem, A. A., Fajrina, H. R., Junus, K. M., ... Ayuningtyas, D. (2016). Integrated Hospital Information System Architecture Design in Indonesia. In T. Iyamu & A. Tatnall (Eds.), *Maximizing Healthcare Delivery and Management through Technology Integration* (pp. 207–236). Hershey, PA: IGI Global. doi:10.4018/978-1-4666-9446-0.ch013

Hartman, A., & Brown, S. (2017). Synergism through Therapeutic Visual Arts. In V. Bryan & J. Bird (Eds.), *Healthcare Community Synergism between Patients, Practitioners, and Researchers* (pp. 29–48). Hershey, PA: IGI Global. doi:10.4018/978-1-5225-0640-9.ch002

Horner, V., & Coleman, A. (2016). Strengthening Implementation of Guidelines at Primary Health Care. In T. Iyamu & A. Tatnall (Eds.), *Maximizing Healthcare Delivery and Management through Technology Integration* (pp. 133–151). Hershey, PA: IGI Global. doi:10.4018/978-1-4666-9446-0.ch009

Høstgaard, A. M. (2016). Constructive eHealth Evaluation: Involving the End-User. In A. Dwivedi (Ed.), *Reshaping Medical Practice and Care with Health Information Systems* (pp. 44–86). Hershey, PA: IGI Global. doi:10.4018/978-1-4666-9870-3.ch003

Iltchev, P., Śliwczyński, A., Szynkiewicz, P., & Marczak, M. (2016). Mobile Health Applications Assisting Patients with Chronic Diseases: Examples from Asthma Care. In A. Moumtzoglou (Ed.), *M-Health Innovations for Patient-Centered Care* (pp. 170–196). Hershey, PA: IGI Global. doi:10.4018/978-1-4666-9861-1.ch009

Iyamu, T., & Mkhomazi, S. S. (2016). Managing Knowledge towards Enabling Healthcare Service Delivery. In T. Iyamu & A. Tatnall (Eds.), *Maximizing Healthcare Delivery and Management through Technology Integration* (pp. 15–26). Hershey, PA: IGI Global. doi:10.4018/978-1-4666-9446-0.ch002

Karon, R. (2016). Utilisation of Health Information Systems for Service Delivery in the Namibian Environment. In T. Iyamu & A. Tatnall (Eds.), *Maximizing Healthcare Delivery and Management through Technology Integration* (pp. 169–183). Hershey, PA: IGI Global. doi:10.4018/978-1-4666-9446-0.ch011

Kasemsap, K. (2017). Telemedicine and Electronic Health: Issues and Implications in Developing Countries. In K. Moahi, K. Bwalya, & P. Sebina (Eds.), *Health Information Systems and the Advancement of Medical Practice in Developing Countries* (pp. 149–167). Hershey, PA: IGI Global. doi:10.4018/978-1-5225-2262-1.ch009

Katuu, S. (2017). Health Information Systems, eHealth Strategy, and the Management of Health Records: The Quest to Transform South Africa's Public Health Sector. In K. Moahi, K. Bwalya, & P. Sebina (Eds.), *Health Information Systems and the Advancement of Medical Practice in Developing Countries* (pp. 237–261). Hershey, PA: IGI Global. doi:10.4018/978-1-5225-2262-1.ch014

Kazandjian, V. A. (2017). We Can Trust without Data, But We Are Accountable Only through Measurement. In A. Moumtzoglou (Ed.), *Design, Development, and Integration of Reliable Electronic Healthcare Platforms* (pp. 255–270). Hershey, PA: IGI Global. doi:10.4018/978-1-5225-1724-5.ch015

Kenski, C. M., & Falcone, J. N. (2017). Humane Education: A Call to Action for Elementary School Students. In V. Bryan & J. Bird (Eds.), *Healthcare Community Synergism between Patients, Practitioners, and Researchers* (pp. 88–105). Hershey, PA: IGI Global. doi:10.4018/978-1-5225-0640-9.ch005

Khumalo, N. B. (2017). "It Has Been Quite a Journey": Experiences and Evolution in Health Information Systems in Zimbabwe. In K. Moahi, K. Bwalya, & P. Sebina (Eds.), *Health Information Systems and the Advancement of Medical Practice in Developing Countries* (pp. 193–207). Hershey, PA: IGI Global. doi:10.4018/978-1-5225-2262-1.ch012

King, B. M., Barry, C. D., Bamdas, J. A., Bronner, K., & Edwards, K. A. (2017). HeartMath®: A University Initiative. In V. Bryan & J. Bird (Eds.), *Healthcare Community Synergism between Patients, Practitioners, and Researchers* (pp. 49–64). Hershey, PA: IGI Global. doi:10.4018/978-1-5225-0640-9.ch003

Kipanyula, M. J., Sanga, C. A., Geofrey, A. M., & Fue, K. G. (2016). On Piloting Web-Based Rabies Surveillance System for Humans and Animals: Web-Based Rabies Surveillance System. In T. Iyamu & A. Tatnall (Eds.), *Maximizing Healthcare Delivery and Management through Technology Integration* (pp. 305–323). Hershey, PA: IGI Global. doi:10.4018/978-1-4666-9446-0.ch017

Komendziński, T., Mikołajewska, E., & Mikołajewski, D. (2018). Cross-Cultural Decision-Making in Healthcare: Theory and Practical Application in Real Clinical Conditions. In A. Rosiek-Kryszewska & K. Leksowski (Eds.), *Healthcare Administration for Patient Safety and Engagement* (pp. 276–298). Hershey, PA: IGI Global. doi:10.4018/978-1-5225-3946-9.ch015

Koumaditis, K., & Themistocleous, M. (2016). SOA Governance in Healthcare: Beyond Early Ideas to a Structured Framework. In A. Dwivedi (Ed.), *Reshaping Medical Practice and Care with Health Information Systems* (pp. 266–286). Hershey, PA: IGI Global. doi:10.4018/978-1-4666-9870-3.ch009

Koumpouros, Y., & Georgoulas, A. (2016). mHealth R&D Activities in Europe. In A. Moumtzoglou (Ed.), M-Health Innovations for Patient-Centered Care (pp. 20-51). Hershey, PA: IGI Global. doi:10.4018/978-1-4666-9861-1.ch002

Liberska, H. (2018). Building a Sense of Security in a Patient: A Psychological Perspective. In A. Rosiek-Kryszewska & K. Leksowski (Eds.), *Healthcare Administration for Patient Safety and Engagement* (pp. 145–173). Hershey, PA: IGI Global. doi:10.4018/978-1-5225-3946-9.ch008

Lidia, B., Federica, G., & Maria, V. E. (2016). The Patient-Centered Medicine as the Theoretical Framework for Patient Engagement. In G. Graffigna (Ed.), *Promoting Patient Engagement and Participation for Effective Healthcare Reform* (pp. 25–39). Hershey, PA: IGI Global. doi:10.4018/978-1-4666-9992-2.ch002

Lin, C., Jalleh, G., & Huang, Y. (2016). Evaluating and Managing Electronic Commerce and Outsourcing Projects in Hospitals. In A. Dwivedi (Ed.), *Reshaping Medical Practice and Care with Health Information Systems* (pp. 132–172). Hershey, PA: IGI Global. doi:10.4018/978-1-4666-9870-3.ch005

Magnavita, N. (2016). Engagement in Health and Safety at the Workplace: A New Role for the Occupational Health Physician. In G. Graffigna (Ed.), *Promoting Patient Engagement and Participation for Effective Healthcare Reform* (pp. 265–289). Hershey, PA: IGI Global. doi:10.4018/978-1-4666-9992-2.ch013

Malanga, D. F. (2017). Implementation of Mobile Health Initiatives in Malawi: Current Status, Issues, and Challenges. In K. Moahi, K. Bwalya, & P. Sebina (Eds.), *Health Information Systems and the Advancement of Medical Practice in Developing Countries* (pp. 115–128). Hershey, PA: IGI Global. doi:10.4018/978-1-5225-2262-1.ch007

Manzoor, A. (2016). RFID Applications in Healthcare-State-of-the-Art and Future Trends. In T. Iyamu & A. Tatnall (Eds.), *Maximizing Healthcare Delivery and Management through Technology Integration* (pp. 184–206). Hershey, PA: IGI Global. doi:10.4018/978-1-4666-9446-0.ch012

Mazzoni, D., & Alberici, A. I. (2016). Why do Patients Protest? Collective Action Processes in People with Chronic Illnesses: A Psychosocial Perspective. In G. Graffigna (Ed.), *Promoting Patient Engagement and Participation for Effective Healthcare Reform* (pp. 128–150). Hershey, PA: IGI Global. doi:10.4018/978-1-4666-9992-2.ch007

Mehta, P. (2017). Framework of Indian Healthcare System and its Challenges: An Insight. In V. Bryan & J. Bird (Eds.), *Healthcare Community Synergism between Patients, Practitioners, and Researchers* (pp. 247–271). Hershey, PA: IGI Global. doi:10.4018/978-1-5225-0640-9.ch011

Mendes, D., Lopes, M., Romão, A., & Rodrigues, I. P. (2017). Healthcare Computer Reasoning Addressing Chronically Ill Societies Using IoT: Deep Learning AI to the Rescue of Home-Based Healthcare. In A. Moumtzoglou (Ed.), *Design, Development, and Integration of Reliable Electronic Healthcare Platforms* (pp. 32–48). Hershey, PA: IGI Global. doi:10.4018/978-1-5225-1724-5.ch002

Metelmann, B., & Metelmann, C. (2016). M-Health in Prehospital Emergency Medicine: Experiences from the EU funded Project LiveCity. In A. Moumtzoglou (Ed.), *M-Health Innovations for Patient-Centered Care* (pp. 197–212). Hershey, PA: IGI Global. doi:10.4018/978-1-4666-9861-1.ch010

Miglioretti, M., Mariani, F., & Vecchio, L. (2016). Could Patient Engagement Promote a Health System Free From Malpractice Litigation Risk? In G. Graffigna (Ed.), *Promoting Patient Engagement and Participation for Effective Healthcare Reform* (pp. 240–264). Hershey, PA: IGI Global. doi:10.4018/978-1-4666-9992-2.ch012

Misra, R. (2016). The Benefits and Challenges of Using Mobile-Based Tools in Self-Management and Care. In A. Dwivedi (Ed.), *Reshaping Medical Practice and Care with Health Information Systems* (pp. 1–13). Hershey, PA: IGI Global. doi:10.4018/978-1-4666-9870-3.ch001

Moahi, K. H. (2017). Big Data and Healthcare: Implications for Medical and Health Care in Low Resource Countries. In K. Moahi, K. Bwalya, & P. Sebina (Eds.), *Health Information Systems and the Advancement of Medical Practice in Developing Countries* (pp. 14–32). Hershey, PA: IGI Global. doi:10.4018/978-1-5225-2262-1.ch002

Moahi, K. H., & Bwalya, K. J. (2017). Knowledge Sharing for Healthcare and Medicine in Developing Countries: Opportunities, Issues, and Experiences. In K. Moahi, K. Bwalya, & P. Sebina (Eds.), *Health Information Systems and the Advancement of Medical Practice in Developing Countries* (pp. 60–77). Hershey, PA: IGI Global. doi:10.4018/978-1-5225-2262-1.ch004

Moghimi, H., Wickramasinghe, N., & Schaffer, J. L. (2016). Intelligent Risk Detection in Healthcare Contexts of Hip and Knee Athroplasty and Paediatric Congenital Heart Disease. In T. Iyamu & A. Tatnall (Eds.), *Maximizing Healthcare Delivery and Management through Technology Integration* (pp. 1–14). Hershey, PA: IGI Global. doi:10.4018/978-1-4666-9446-0.ch001

Moumtzoglou, A. (2017). Digital Medicine: The Quality Standpoint. In A. Moumtzoglou (Ed.), *Design, Development, and Integration of Reliable Electronic Healthcare Platforms* (pp. 179–195). Hershey, PA: IGI Global. doi:10.4018/978-1-5225-1724-5.ch011

Moumtzoglou, A., & Pouliakis, A. (2017). Population Health Management and Cervical Cancer Screening Programs: Roadmap, Design, and Implementation of a Supporting IT System. In A. Moumtzoglou (Ed.), *Design, Development, and Integration of Reliable Electronic Healthcare Platforms* (pp. 1–31). Hershey, PA: IGI Global. doi:10.4018/978-1-5225-1724-5.ch001

Moumtzoglou, A. S. (2016). Tailored M-Health Communication in Patient-Centered Care. In A. Moumtzoglou (Ed.), *M-Health Innovations for Patient-Centered Care* (pp. 319–340). Hershey, PA: IGI Global. doi:10.4018/978-1-4666-9861-1.ch016

Moumtzoglou, A. S. (2016). The Nexus of M-Health and Self-Efficacy. In A. Moumtzoglou (Ed.), *M-Health Innovations for Patient-Centered Care* (pp. 341–365). Hershey, PA: IGI Global. doi:10.4018/978-1-4666-9861-1.ch017

Mreła, A., & Sokołov, O. (2018). Formal Methods for Assessing Patient Satisfaction in a Patient-Doctor Relationship. In A. Rosiek-Kryszewska & K. Leksowski (Eds.), *Healthcare Administration for Patient Safety and Engagement* (pp. 201–219). Hershey, PA: IGI Global. doi:10.4018/978-1-5225-3946-9.ch011

Mularska-Kucharek, M. (2018). Social Capital and Subjective Quality of Life. In A. Rosiek-Kryszewska & K. Leksowski (Eds.), *Healthcare Administration for Patient Safety and Engagement* (pp. 174–185). Hershey, PA: IGI Global. doi:10.4018/978-1-5225-3946-9.ch009

Ndlovu, K., Mauco, K. L., & Littman-Quinn, R. (2017). Telemedicine in Low Resource Settings: A Case for Botswana. In K. Moahi, K. Bwalya, & P. Sebina (Eds.), *Health Information Systems and the Advancement of Medical Practice in Developing Countries* (pp. 129–148). Hershey, PA: IGI Global. doi:10.4018/978-1-5225-2262-1.ch008

Nemutanzhela, P., & Iyamu, T. (2016). Introducing Mobile Device for Health Services: The Semantics of Language Translation. In T. Iyamu & A. Tatnall (Eds.), *Maximizing Healthcare Delivery and Management through Technology Integration* (pp. 101–112). Hershey, PA: IGI Global. doi:10.4018/978-1-4666-9446-0.ch007

Nishimura, S., & Scott, D. J. (2016). Waseda University's E-School: 10 Years of E-Education in Japan. In A. Dwivedi (Ed.), *Reshaping Medical Practice and Care with Health Information Systems* (pp. 173–204). Hershey, PA: IGI Global. doi:10.4018/978-1-4666-9870-3.ch006

Noordin, M. F., Arshad, A., & Othman, R. (2017). KIIPF - An Integrated Inter-Operable Knowledge Management Process Framework for Healthcare: Implementation in Pakistani Healthcare Industry. *Journal of Cases on Information Technology*, *19*(3), 24–41. doi:10.4018/JCIT.2017070103

Pasternak, A. (2018). Building Relationships Within a Therapeutic Team. In A. Rosiek-Kryszewska & K. Leksowski (Eds.), *Healthcare Administration for Patient Safety and Engagement* (pp. 220–243). Hershey, PA: IGI Global. doi:10.4018/978-1-5225-3946-9.ch012

Pieczka, B. (2018). Management of Risk and Adverse Events in Medical Entities. In A. Rosiek-Kryszewska & K. Leksowski (Eds.), *Healthcare Administration for Patient Safety and Engagement* (pp. 31–46). Hershey, PA: IGI Global. doi:10.4018/978-1-5225-3946-9.ch003

Pomares-Quimbaya, A., González, R. A., Sierra, A., Daza, J. C., Muñoz, O., García, A., ... Bohórquez, W. R. (2017). ICT for Enabling the Quality Evaluation of Health Care Services: A Case Study in a General Hospital. In A. Moumtzoglou (Ed.), *Design, Development, and Integration of Reliable Electronic Healthcare Platforms* (pp. 196–210). Hershey, PA: IGI Global. doi:10.4018/978-1-5225-1724-5.ch012

Pouliakis, A., Archondakis, S., Margari, N., & Karakitsos, P. (2016). From Telecytology to Mobile Cytopathology: Past, Present, and Future. In A. Moumtzoglou (Ed.), *M-Health Innovations for Patient-Centered Care* (pp. 240–261). Hershey, PA: IGI Global. doi:10.4018/978-1-4666-9861-1.ch012

Provenzi, L., Borgatti, R., & Montirosso, R. (2016). The Light Side of Preterm Behavioral Epigenetics: An Epigenetic Perspective on Caregiver Engagement. In G. Graffigna (Ed.), *Promoting Patient Engagement and Participation for Effective Healthcare Reform* (pp. 107–127). Hershey, PA: IGI Global. doi:10.4018/978-1-4666-9992-2.ch006

Rodrigues, P. M., Freitas, D., Teixeira, J. P., Alves, D., & Garrett, C. (2017). Early Detection of Electroencephalogram Temporal Events in Alzheimer's Disease. In A. Moumtzoglou (Ed.), *Design, Development, and Integration of Reliable Electronic Healthcare Platforms* (pp. 112–131). Hershey, PA: IGI Global. doi:10.4018/978-1-5225-1724-5.ch007

Rosiek, A. (2018). The Assessment of Actions of the Environment and the Impact of Preventive Medicine for Public Health in Poland. In A. Rosiek-Kryszewska & K. Leksowski (Eds.), *Healthcare Administration for Patient Safety and Engagement* (pp. 106–119). Hershey, PA: IGI Global. doi:10.4018/978-1-5225-3946-9.ch006

Rosiek, A., & Rosiek-Kryszewska, A. (2018). Managed Healthcare: Doctor Life Satisfaction and Its Impact on the Process of Communicating With the Patient. In A. Rosiek-Kryszewska & K. Leksowski (Eds.), *Healthcare Administration for Patient Safety and Engagement* (pp. 244–261). Hershey, PA: IGI Global. doi:10.4018/978-1-5225-3946-9.ch013

Rosiek-Kryszewska, A., & Rosiek, A. (2018). The Impact of Management and Leadership Roles in Building Competitive Healthcare Units. In A. Rosiek-Kryszewska & K. Leksowski (Eds.), *Healthcare Administration for Patient Safety and Engagement* (pp. 13–30). Hershey, PA: IGI Global. doi:10.4018/978-1-5225-3946-9.ch002

Rosiek-Kryszewska, A., & Rosiek, A. (2018). The Involvement of the Patient and his Perspective Evaluation of the Quality of Healthcare. In A. Rosiek-Kryszewska & K. Leksowski (Eds.), *Healthcare Administration for Patient Safety and Engagement* (pp. 121–144). Hershey, PA: IGI Global. doi:10.4018/978-1-5225-3946-9.ch007

Ross, D. B., Exposito, J. A., & Kennedy, T. (2017). Stress and Its Relationship to Leadership and a Healthy Workplace Culture. In V. Bryan & J. Bird (Eds.), *Healthcare Community Synergism between Patients, Practitioners, and Researchers* (pp. 213–246). Hershey, PA: IGI Global. doi:10.4018/978-1-5225-0640-9.ch010

Sagahyroon, A. (2016). mHealth: Sleeping Disorders Diagnosis. In A. Moumtzoglou (Ed.), M-Health Innovations for Patient-Centered Care (pp. 115-125). Hershey, PA: IGI Global. doi:10.4018/978-1-4666-9861-1.ch006

Sam, S. (2017). Mobile Phones and Expanding Human Capabilities in Plural Health Systems. In K. Moahi, K. Bwalya, & P. Sebina (Eds.), *Health Information Systems and the Advancement of Medical Practice in Developing Countries* (pp. 93–114). Hershey, PA: IGI Global. doi:10.4018/978-1-5225-2262-1.ch006

Sarkar, B. K. (2017). Big Data and Healthcare Data: A Survey. *International Journal of Knowledge-Based Organizations, 7*(4), 50–77. doi:10.4018/IJKBO.2017100104

Sebina, P. M., & Grand, B. (2017). Records Management and Open Data in Healthcare Provision in Africa: Reflections and Lessons for Botswana. In K. Moahi, K. Bwalya, & P. Sebina (Eds.), *Health Information Systems and the Advancement of Medical Practice in Developing Countries* (pp. 1–13). Hershey, PA: IGI Global. doi:10.4018/978-1-5225-2262-1.ch001

Shaanika, I. N. (2016). Human Interaction in the Use of Health Information Systems: A Case of a Developing Country. In T. Iyamu & A. Tatnall (Eds.), *Maximizing Healthcare Delivery and Management through Technology Integration* (pp. 257–269). Hershey, PA: IGI Global. doi:10.4018/978-1-4666-9446-0.ch015

Shi, J., Erdem, E., & Liu, H. (2016). Expanding Role of Telephone Systems in Healthcare: Developments and Opportunities. In A. Dwivedi (Ed.), *Reshaping Medical Practice and Care with Health Information Systems* (pp. 87–131). Hershey, PA: IGI Global. doi:10.4018/978-1-4666-9870-3.ch004

Sielski, Ł., & Soczywko, J. (2018). The Physiotherapist as a Health Educator. In A. Rosiek-Kryszewska & K. Leksowski (Eds.), *Healthcare Administration for Patient Safety and Engagement* (pp. 262–275). Hershey, PA: IGI Global. doi:10.4018/978-1-5225-3946-9.ch014

Soczywko, J., & Rutkowska, D. (2018). The Patient/Provider Relationship in Emergency Medicine: Organization, Communication, and Understanding. In A. Rosiek-Kryszewska & K. Leksowski (Eds.), *Healthcare Administration for Patient Safety and Engagement* (pp. 74–105). Hershey, PA: IGI Global. doi:10.4018/978-1-5225-3946-9.ch005

Sourial, M., Bamdas, J. A., Constanzo, A., & Ishak, M. E. (2017). A Need for Greater Collaboration: Initiatives to Improve Transitions of Care. In V. Bryan & J. Bird (Eds.), *Healthcare Community Synergism between Patients, Practitioners, and Researchers* (pp. 65–87). Hershey, PA: IGI Global. doi:10.4018/978-1-5225-0640-9.ch004

Spinelli, R., & Benevolo, C. (2016). From Healthcare Services to E-Health Applications: A Delivery System-Based Taxonomy. In A. Dwivedi (Ed.), *Reshaping Medical Practice and Care with Health Information Systems* (pp. 205–245). Hershey, PA: IGI Global. doi:10.4018/978-1-4666-9870-3.ch007

Stavros, A., Vavoulidis, E., & Nasioutziki, M. (2016). The Use of Mobile Health Applications for Quality Control and Accreditational Purposes in a Cytopathology Laboratory. In A. Moumtzoglou (Ed.), *M-Health Innovations for Patient-Centered Care* (pp. 262–283). Hershey, PA: IGI Global. doi:10.4018/978-1-4666-9861-1.ch013

Tamposis, I., Pouliakis, A., Fezoulidis, I., & Karakitsos, P. (2016). Mobile Platforms Supporting Health Professionals: Need, Technical Requirements, and Applications. In A. Moumtzoglou (Ed.), *M-Health Innovations for Patient-Centered Care* (pp. 91–114). Hershey, PA: IGI Global. doi:10.4018/978-1-4666-9861-1.ch005

Tanzariello, M., Bucci, S., Ricciardi, W., & Giulio de Belvis, A. (2016). Accountability and Public Reporting: Publication of Performance to Improve Quality. In G. Graffigna (Ed.), *Promoting Patient Engagement and Participation for Effective Healthcare Reform* (pp. 215–239). Hershey, PA: IGI Global. doi:10.4018/978-1-4666-9992-2.ch011

Taweel, A. (2016). Semantic Interoperability-Enabled Architecture for Connected Health Services. In A. Dwivedi (Ed.), *Reshaping Medical Practice and Care with Health Information Systems* (pp. 246–265). Hershey, PA: IGI Global. doi:10.4018/978-1-4666-9870-3.ch008

Teixeira, J. P., Fernandes, M. G., & Costa, R. A. (2017). Automatic Determination of Pauses in Speech for Classification of Stuttering Disorder. In A. Moumtzoglou (Ed.), *Design, Development, and Integration of Reliable Electronic Healthcare Platforms* (pp. 132–149). Hershey, PA: IGI Global. doi:10.4018/978-1-5225-1724-5.ch008

Tiago, M. T., Tiago, F., Amaral, F. E., & Silva, S. (2016). Healthy 3.0: Healthcare Digital Dimensions. In A. Dwivedi (Ed.), *Reshaping Medical Practice and Care with Health Information Systems* (pp. 287–322). Hershey, PA: IGI Global. doi:10.4018/978-1-4666-9870-3.ch010

Tshiamo, W. B., Kgositau, M., & Magowe, M. (2017). Use of Information and Communication Technology by Health Care Providers for Continuing Professional Development in Botswana. In K. Moahi, K. Bwalya, & P. Sebina (Eds.), *Health Information Systems and the Advancement of Medical Practice in Developing Countries* (pp. 181–192). Hershey, PA: IGI Global. doi:10.4018/978-1-5225-2262-1.ch011

Unnithan, C., & Tatnall, A. (2016). Radio Frequency Identification Technology in an Australian Regional Hospital: An Innovation Translation Experience with ANT. In T. Iyamu & A. Tatnall (Eds.), *Maximizing Healthcare Delivery and Management through Technology Integration* (pp. 76–100). Hershey, PA: IGI Global. doi:10.4018/978-1-4666-9446-0.ch006

Unwin, D. W., Sanzogni, L., & Sandhu, K. (2017). Developing and Measuring the Business Case for Health Information Technology. In K. Moahi, K. Bwalya, & P. Sebina (Eds.), *Health Information Systems and the Advancement of Medical Practice in Developing Countries* (pp. 262–290). Hershey, PA: IGI Global. doi:10.4018/978-1-5225-2262-1.ch015

Usher, W. (2017). E-Health: Modern Communication Technology Platforms for Accessing Health Information. In A. Moumtzoglou (Ed.), *Design, Development, and Integration of Reliable Electronic Healthcare Platforms* (pp. 49–71). Hershey, PA: IGI Global. doi:10.4018/978-1-5225-1724-5.ch003

Vaz, N. F. (2018). Patient Satisfaction. In A. Rosiek-Kryszewska & K. Leksowski (Eds.), *Healthcare Administration for Patient Safety and Engagement* (pp. 186–200). Hershey, PA: IGI Global. doi:10.4018/978-1-5225-3946-9.ch010

Vezyridis, P., Timmons, S., & Wharrad, H. (2016). Lessons Learned from the Implementation of an Emergency Department Information System. In T. Iyamu & A. Tatnall (Eds.), *Maximizing Healthcare Delivery and Management through Technology Integration* (pp. 237–256). Hershey, PA: IGI Global. doi:10.4018/978-1-4666-9446-0.ch014

Vlachopapadopoulou, E., & Fotiadis, D. I. (2016). The Contribution of mHealth in the Care of Obese Pediatric Patients. In A. Moumtzoglou (Ed.), *M-Health Innovations for Patient-Centered Care* (pp. 126–146). Hershey, PA: IGI Global. doi:10.4018/978-1-4666-9861-1.ch007

Waegemann, C. P. (2016). mHealth: History, Analysis, and Implementation. In A. Moumtzoglou (Ed.), M-Health Innovations for Patient-Centered Care (pp. 1-19). Hershey, PA: IGI Global. doi:10.4018/978-1-4666-9861-1.ch001

Weiss-Randall, D. N. (2017). The Role of Self-Efficacy and Aging in Managing Disease. In V. Bryan & J. Bird (Eds.), *Healthcare Community Synergism between Patients, Practitioners, and Researchers* (pp. 176–212). Hershey, PA: IGI Global. doi:10.4018/978-1-5225-0640-9.ch009

Wickramasinghe, N., Troshani, I., & Goldberg, S. (2016). A Transaction Cost Economics Perspective for Pervasive Technology. In A. Dwivedi (Ed.), *Reshaping Medical Practice and Care with Health Information Systems* (pp. 14–43). Hershey, PA: IGI Global. doi:10.4018/978-1-4666-9870-3.ch002

Wójcik, A. (2018). The Impact of the Attitude of Medical Staff From Burnout on the Level of Ongoing Medical Services. In A. Rosiek-Kryszewska & K. Leksowski (Eds.), *Healthcare Administration for Patient Safety and Engagement* (pp. 47–73). Hershey, PA: IGI Global. doi:10.4018/978-1-5225-3946-9.ch004

Yu, B., Wijesekera, D., & Costa, P. C. (2017). Informed Consent in Healthcare: A Study Case of Genetic Services. In A. Moumtzoglou (Ed.), *Design, Development, and Integration of Reliable Electronic Healthcare Platforms* (pp. 211–242). Hershey, PA: IGI Global. doi:10.4018/978-1-5225-1724-5.ch013

Zimeras, S. (2016). Computer Virus Models and Analysis in M-Health IT Systems: Computer Virus Models. In A. Moumtzoglou (Ed.), *M-Health Innovations for Patient-Centered Care* (pp. 284–297). Hershey, PA: IGI Global. doi:10.4018/978-1-4666-9861-1.ch014

Zimeras, S. (2017). Surface Segmentation: The Case of Bronchus Anatomical Structure. In A. Moumtzoglou (Ed.), *Design, Development, and Integration of Reliable Electronic Healthcare Platforms* (pp. 150–159). Hershey, PA: IGI Global. doi:10.4018/978-1-5225-1724-5.ch009

Ziminski, T. B., Demurjian, S. A., Sanzi, E., & Agresta, T. (2016). Toward Integrating Healthcare Data and Systems: A Study of Architectural Alternatives. In T. Iyamu & A. Tatnall (Eds.), *Maximizing Healthcare Delivery and Management through Technology Integration* (pp. 270–304). Hershey, PA: IGI Global. doi:10.4018/978-1-4666-9446-0.ch016

About the Author

Francesca Costanza holds an international PhD in Model Based Public Planning, Policy Design and Management at the University of Palermo (Italy), a MD in Business Economics and Administration and a Msc in Healthcare Management. She was guest researcher at the universities of Bergen and Nijmegen and also conducted EU funded research at the Italian National Council of Research. She is currently lecturer of 'Corporate groups and consolidated financial statements' at LUMSA University (Palermo). Her research interests are: public management, healthcare management, value co-creation, entrepreneurship and digital entrepreneurship, sustainable tourism.

Index

P

Q

R

S

U

V

www.ingramcontent.com/pod-product-compliance
Lightning Source LLC
LaVergne TN
LVHW080853300926
849162LV00003B/414
* 9 7 8 1 7 9 9 8 2 6 5 3 8 *